American

Narcan

Naloxone & Heroin-Fentanyl associated Mortality

35th Circuit Drug Court Shiawassee County

Bay County Health Department

The Office of the Deputy Chief Medical Examiner &

Recovery Pathways Behavioral Health Institute

Queen of Angels Women's Detox Residence

Morrone & Morrone

Copyright © 2017 by William Morrone

Funding and the advisory board are the same person and he/she hates committees and meetings.

Working for hospitals and medical schools left me feeling numb and embalmed, because every organization admitted there was a heroin overdose problem but they turned away citing some line about, "there's no money in it" or "it's not primary care." Corporations were supposed to be this way but not medical schools and surely not hospitals.

I am unrepentant and the whole system is broken.

This book was designed to read on an iPhone or a Galaxy type screen.

https://www.youtube.com/watch?v=yKmOZR6WefU

https://www.youtube.com/watch?v=u95KzSlFSKQ

https://www.youtube.com/watch?v=pbNwnwoHapI&sns=em

ISBN-13:   978-0-9892263-18

American Narcan is a call to arms.

Who is the Target?

Parents, **P**roviders, **P**artners and/or **P**eople are at risk if they have opioids in the house with children and teens.

The overarching goal of **American Narcan** is to offer public health data, addiction medicine policy and commentary to support informed evidence-based trainings on the safe and effective use. Opinion is translated on the prescribing or distribution of the naloxone family of medications in the treatment of substance use disorder, heroin overdose and opioid addiction.

Naloxone treatment is FDA approved to be used by family members or caregivers to treat persons unknown or suspected to have had an opioid overdose.

Naloxone is an answer. It needs to be in every home.

Our focus is to reach providers and diverse professions including first responders, physicians, nurses, dentists, physician assistants, pharmacists, school principals, coaches, educators, law enforcement, clergy, criminal justice staff, legislators, legislative consultants, talk show hosts, news producers, health program administrators, social workers, spouses and **parents.**

There will be people that are opioid dependent that are not addicted but severe chronic pain patients with chronic disease or high dose opioids. These people are also at risk. Naloxone is an answer.

Heroin and opioid overdose deaths are touching more people and American families than any fatal public health problem in 100 years. Naloxone is an answer.

No agency has an accurate number of heroin deaths. Numbers (federal and state) are far too low.

Res Ipsa Locquitur

The import of a thing or situation is obvious. It effectively shifts the burden of proof to the defendant.

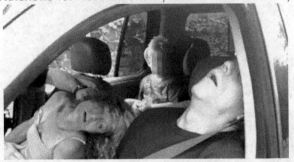

Photo posted on Police Department website.

Parents made the news overdosing in front of their kids. Opioid overdose death numbers are not reported real-time. The news and states reports E. coli in your lakes, smog in your air, flash floods in your land and flu in your schools. Heroin is killing more people daily under the age of 24 than flu, floods and smog. Dinosaurs and stigma abound. Are you defenseless?

Naloxone is an answer. *American Narcan* is an infographopedia.

American Narcan is your call to arms. The reader must rethink first responder. Our distinctness is to expand first responder and sometimes push your comfort level right up to your comfort limit.

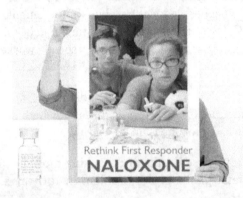

American Narcan cannot be a Gray's Anatomy or Guyton's Physiology type book. ***American Narcan*** has to be born and delivered in the same assumption that Martin Luther used 500 years ago. **Go to the people.**

Drug addiction has many pathways to recovery but opioid overdose death only has one pathway back to rescue and reversal. That is naloxone.

We have greater than 1,000,000 providers in a healthcare system that directly or indirectly created a decade of addiction in the fog of incomplete monitoring, misguided "utilization" and inaccurate engagement.

4

Drug dealers have put more marketing strategy into feedback from public need than hospital systems.

When our police save more people from overdose than our doctors I am ashamed that more providers did not stand in the gap.

"And I sought for a man among them, that should make up the hedge, and stand in the gap before me for the land, that I should not destroy it: but I found none."

Ezekiel 22:30

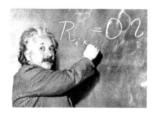

Pancakes w/ Einstein Publishing - Bay City, MI

TABLE OF CONTENTS

Editor:

William R. Morrone, DO MS MPH

Fellow – American Osteopathic Academy of Addiction Medicine

Past President, Michigan Society of Addiction Medicine; Bay County – Deputy Chief Medical Examiner

Medical Director, Recovery Pathways Behavioral Health Institute (RPBHI)

Medical Director, Queen of Angels Detox-Holy Cross Services

My Teachers:

Victoria Tutag Lehr, Pharm D

Professor, Eugene Applebaum College of Pharmacy, Wayne State University

Pamela Lynch, LMSW, CAADC

Northern Lakes Community Mental Health T City, Grand Valley State University, Grand Rapids, MI, Harm Reduction Michigan

Carl Christensen, MD, PhD

Fellow – American Society of Addiction Medicine

Past President, Michigan Society of Addiction Medicine; Medical Director, Christensen Recovery

Medical Director, Health Professional Recovery

Naloxone Preface

What is naloxone? Naloxone is an opioid *antagonist medication.* Naloxone reverses opioid overdose.

Naloxone hydrochloride is a generic (I.V., I.M., & S.C.), low-cost, non-narcotic opioid antagonist that blocks the brain cell receptors activated by opioids like heroin, oxycodone, hydrocodone and other opioids.

Naloxone is not psychoative, has no poential for abuse and side effects are rare. Naloxone is used both in the U.S. and abroad. The mean serum half - life has been shown to range from 30 to 81 minutes, necessitating repeat dosing.

Naloxone is metabolized by the liver. Its major metabolites have been naloxone-3-glucuronide and *noroxymorphone.*

In our world, science, medicine, teaching, law, criminal justice investigation and toxicology explain mystery and discover truth. Sometimes making complex medical facts into simple honest sound bites is really the only true justice. Teaching and knowledge are the only weapons against fear and ignorance.

Does your doctor speak naloxone? Maybe 2-3% do.

Naloxone is arguably the most important medicine in the Americas. Healthcare systems, hospitals, community mental health and medical schools cannot respond to heroin because they have not been engaged. They project stigma.

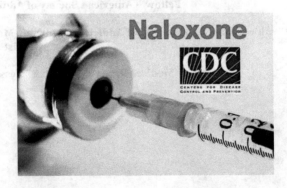

Naloxone

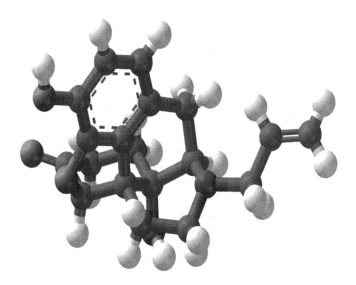

Sold under the brand name Narcan or Evzio, naloxone is a fast- acting drug that, when administered during an overdose, blocks the effects of opioids on the brain and restores breathing within two to three minutes of administration.

Approved by the FDA in 1971, naloxone has been used safely and effectively for over 4 decades in ambulances and emergency rooms across America.

In America and around the world, naloxone distribution programs are currently training potential overdose witnesses to correctly recognize an overdose and administer the drug, greatly reducing the risk of accidental death.

The CDC has recognized co-prescribed naloxone in their 2016 guidelines as an effort to reduce death in high risk pain populations that include advanced age, chronic disease and doses that exceed 50 morphine milli-equivalents (MME) and/or co-medication with benzodiazepines.

The larger portion to benefit from naloxone is 3rd party prescribing and naloxone distribution designed to reduce heroin overdose deaths. Drug overdose deaths are at an all-time high in America.

There are at least two ways to view the 3rd party:

A. A *"third-party"* (3rd party) means a party that is not directly controlled by either the provider (1st party) or the patient/customer (2nd party) in a clinical/business transaction. The third party is considered independent from the other two, because not all control is vested in that connection. There can be multiple third-party sources with respect to a given clinical/business transaction, between the first and second parties.

B. 1st party prescribing is directly to the patient (party) in front of you.

2nd party prescribing is to the patient (party) geographically next to the communicating responsible party in front of you.

3rd party prescribing is to a party not present. Your patient (2nd party) participates in a counseling event about the party (3rd party) not present.

1st party prescribing is what every provider learns in school. Prescribing is modified in pediatrics, geriatrics and hospice to 2nd party prescribing. 3rd party prescribing is novel and the only way to interdict in the heroin overdose death epidemic.

Here we are reflecting a model that is more public health and less doctor patient relationship.

Naloxone distribution, also a public health model, is used both in the America and abroad. By providing training on and access to naloxone, overdose prevention and treatment programs have enabled bystanders to save thousands of lives by reversing overdoses.

Why do you need naloxone?

Why does America need naloxone?

52,404 people died of drug overdose in 2015 and we are tracking for 70,000.

Naloxone could have saved 63% of them

It's all about the death curve.

You need American Narcan because you cannot change enough laws or educate enough doctors to change the death curve.

The death curve is also very likely worse than what is reported.

You need American Narcan because lawmakers still just don't get it.

You need American Narcan because your doctor doesn't get it. Heroin is below the radar of state appointed bureaucrats and law makers.

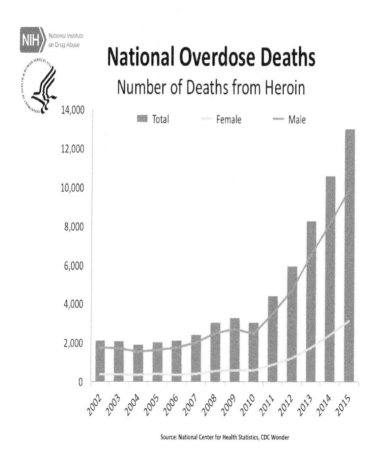

Source: National Center for Health Statistics, CDC Wonder

Despite comprising a smaller user population, there were more treatment admissions to publicly funded facilities for heroin than for any other drug.

Abstinence based therapy and Community Health Centers still have not wrapped their head around the death curve. I walk amoung people weekly that debate whether or not they should support community naloxone.

It's all about the death curve.

Every publically funded facility for heroin treatment or opioid use disorder should be a hub for the distribution or prescribing of naloxone.

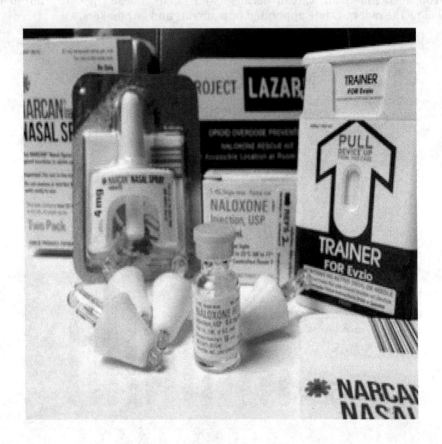

Heroin Preface

What is heroin?

Heroin is not natural. Heroin is a crude preparation of diamorphine. It is a semisynthetic product obtained by *acetylation of morphine*, which occurs as a natural product in opium: the dried latex of certain poppy species (e.g. *Papaver somniferum* L.). Diamorphine, first synthesized in 1847, is used in the treatment of severe pain. Illicit heroin may be smoked, snorted or solubilized with a weak acid and injected.

heroin

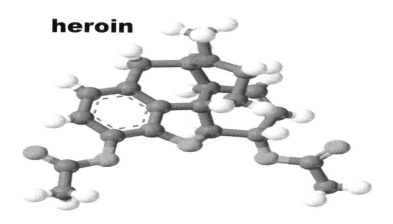

Whereas opium has been smoked since historical times, diamorphine was first synthesised in the late nineteenth century. Heroin is under international control.

Heroin is classified as **Schedule I** in the United States, meaning that the DEA considers it to have no currently accepted medical use and a high potential for abuse.

Drug overdose deaths, including heroin deaths, are at an all-time high in America. Naloxone has to be the core of any strategy not just prescription drug monitoring because heroin is not on drug monitoring software. CDC (2014) noted of the Heroin users since 2000, 75% started on prescription drugs. This may be higher today.

From the New York Times, January 19, 2016:

"Deaths from drug overdoses have jumped in nearly every county across the United States, driven largely by an explosion in addiction to prescription painkillers and **heroin**.

The largest concentrations of overdose deaths were in Appalachia and the Southwest, according to new county-level estimates released by the Centers for Disease Control and Prevention.

The number of these deaths reached a new peak in 2014: 47,055 people, or the equivalent of about 125 Americans every day."

The (2016 newly released data for) 2015 number of drug overdose deaths is worse at 52,404. 2016 data will be available in late 2017 or early 2018. Crude numbers suggest 59,799 but many counties still do not report to the state.

Heroin or Diamorphine, like morphine produces analgesia. It behaves as an **agonist** at a complex group of receptors (the μ, κ and δ subtypes) that are normally acted upon by endogenous peptides known as endorphins. Apart from analgesia, diamorphine produces drowsiness, euphoria and a sense of detachment.

Negative effects include respiratory depression, nausea and vomiting, decreased motility in the gastrointestinal tract, suppression of the cough reflex and hypothermia. Tolerance and physical dependence occur on repeated use. Cessation of use in tolerant subjects leads to characteristic withdrawal symptoms.

Subjective effects following injection are known as 'the rush' and are associated with feelings of warmth and pleasure, followed by a longer period of sedation. Diamorphine is 2–3 times more **potent** than morphine.

Data is conflicted.

CNN (2017) reports that heroin use has increased five fold. The CIA has estimated that in 2015, 66% of the world's supply of heroin came from Afghanistan.

DEA National Threat Drug Assessment states the 79% of America heroin seized is from the Mexican pipeline.

No matter.

Naloxone has been the gold standard treatment for heroin overdoses for four decades.

Heroin Street Price:

The mean retail price of brown heroin continues higher in Nordic countries than the rest of Europe and ranged between EUR 24 (Bulgaria), $25.26 (U.S.) and EUR 143 (Sweden) $150.52 (U.S.) per gram.

The price of white heroin is reported only by a few European countries and ranged between EUR 62.7 (Italy), $66.00 (U.S.) and EUR 249 (Sweden), $262.10 (U.S.) per gram.

Heroin use is not mainstream, at this time. How did it become so proliferative and popular? Decreased access to prescription opioids did not stop people from using opioids. Decreased access caused a transfer to heroin.

People may be addicted to heroin and/or prescription opioids.

The public and the media misalign the word "addiction and addicted" to people that have an ethical treatment plan that an opioid is a responsible regular component.

How can you separate the difference?

ADDICTION in the cultural setting: The addiction concept may linger but official clinical use of the "addiction" word has to be phased out because it has been judged to be pejorative. Washington DC leadership is responsible here. Its days are numbered by appointed leaders and people that Skype. Let me play devil's advocate about terminology.

I have sat in the Friday night open NA (Narcotics Anonymous) meeting at Trinity Episcopal and the word "addict" is embraced. 100 people in the room say "*I am an addict*" sooner or later.

You are going to have a hard time telling them to stop saying addict. The word addict is a source of power and association to people that hug. These people hug really hard. Men hug men and slap backs up between the shoulder blades.

Nobody is afraid to hug a stranger at NA. On the contrary, nobody is hugging on Skype, in the capital or HHS meetings.

Addicts find the need to re-center them self in a brief statement about the past and reaffirmation that we are more than the sum of our failures. The word addict is a critical ingredient. The word addict is a street sign designating firm ground and direction.

The word addict is claimed by people that presented monologues of promise to new people seeking help.

Addict is the term that one ignites their own daily journey of healing and self-discovery.

ADDICTION in the clinical setting: The American Psychiatric Association has introduced the new DSM-V.

Substance use disorders span a wide variety of problems arising from substance use, and cover 11 different criteria:

1. *Taking the substance in larger amounts or for longer than the you meant to*
2. *Wanting to cut down or stop using the substance but not managing to*
3. *Spending a lot of time getting, using, or recovering from use of the substance*
4. *Cravings and urges to use the substance*
5. *Not managing to do what you should at work, home or school, because of substance use*
6. *Continuing to use, even when it causes problems in relationships*
7. *Giving up important social, occupational or recreational activities because of substance use*
8. *Using substances again and again, even when it puts the you in danger*
9. *Continuing to use, even when the you know you have a physical or psychological problem that could have been caused or made worse by the substance*
10. *Needing more of the substance to get the effect you want (tolerance)*
11. *Development of withdrawal symptoms, which can be relieved by taking more of the substance.*

The DSM 5 allows clinicians to specify how severe the substance use disorder is, depending on how many symptoms are identified.

Two or three symptoms indicate a mild substance use disorder, four or five symptoms indicate a moderate substance use disorder, and six or more symptoms indicate a severe substance use disorder.

An absence of DSM-V symptoms during treatment with opioids is generally ethical pain management. This is the goal of mainstream opioid-based pain management.

Heroin use is never considered mainstream because it involves pathways that transgress, federal regulatory approval, an ethical pharmaceutical industry, graduate medical training, human trafficking, organized crime, criminal justice and law enforcement prime directives.

Heroin Use Has INCREASED Among Most Demographic Groups

	2002-2004*	2011-2013*	% CHANGE
SEX			
Male	2.4	3.6	50%
Female	0.8	1.6	100%
AGE, YEARS			
12-17	1.8	1.6	--
18-25	3.5	7.3	109%
26 or older	1.2	1.9	58%
RACE/ETHNICITY			
Non-Hispanic white	1.4	3	114%
Other	2	1.7	--
ANNUAL HOUSEHOLD INCOME			
Less than $20,000	3.4	5.5	62%
$20,000-$49,999	1.3	2.3	77%
$50,000 or more	1	1.6	60%
HEALTH INSURANCE COVERAGE			
None	4.2	6.7	60%
Medicaid	4.3	4.7	--
Private or other	0.8	1.3	63%

Heroin Addiction and Overdose Deaths are Climbing

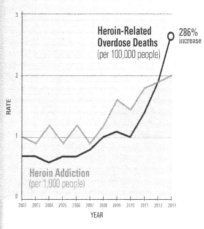

Heroin-Related Overdose Deaths (per 100,000 people) — 286% increase

Heroin Addiction (per 1,000 people)

RATE

YEAR

SOURCES: National Survey on Drug Use and Health (NSDUH), 2002-2013.
National Vital Statistics System, 2002-2013.

Synthetic Opioid Overdose Death Rates

Age-adjusted deaths per 100,000 population for synthetic opioids (excluding methadone, including fentanyl and tramadol) from 2014 to **2015**, by census region of residence

 2.7   5.6 **Northeast***
3,071 Deaths in 2015

 2.0   3.9 **Midwest***
2,548 Deaths in 2015

 1.8   2.8 **South***
3,303 Deaths in 2015

 0.8 0.9 **West***
658 Deaths in 2015

 1.8   3.1 **United States***
9,580 Deaths in 2015

0   1   2   3   4   5   6   7   8

SOURCE: CDC/NCHS, National Vital Statistics System, Mortality. CDC WONDER, Atlanta, GA: US Department of Health and Human Services, CDC; 2016. https://wonder.cdc.gov/.

* Statistically significant at p<0.05 level.

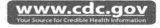
www.cdc.gov
Your Source for Credible Health Information

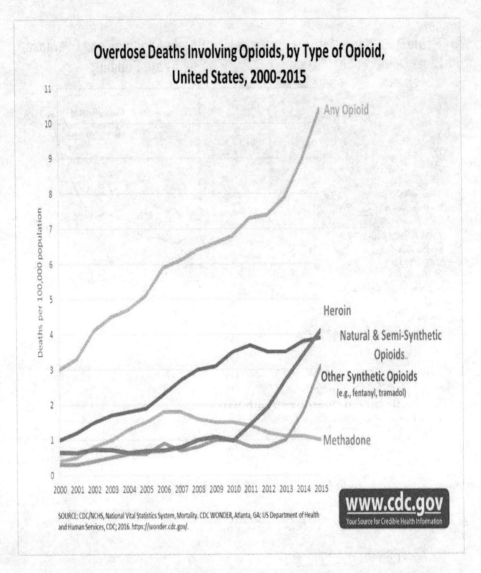

Translated narrative: Heroin and synthetics in America are rising with no sign of slowing down. Prescription (Rx) deaths are leveling out. People and physicians are not better with Rx behavioir. People are cut off and are switching to heroin. Methadone deaths are declining. 2016-2017 over dose death data will be worse than ever.

●●●○○ Verizon 🤳   12:55 PM   🔆 91% 📶▪

cdc.gov

Statistically significant changes in drug overdose death rates involving synthetic opioids (excluding methadone) by select states, United States, 2014 to 2015

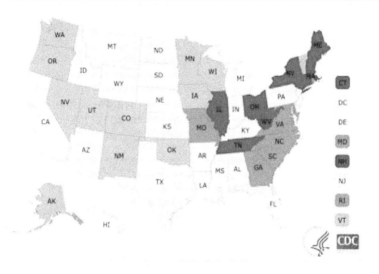

Statistically significant change in rate, 2014-2015

Statistically significant changes in drug overdose death* rates involving synthetic opioids[†] (excluding methadone) by select states,[††] United States, 2014 to 2015.

Note: Rate comparisons between states should not be made due to variations in reporting across states.

* Deaths are classified using the International Classification of Diseases, Tenth Revision (ICD-10). Drug overdose deaths are identified using underlying cause-of-death codes X40-X44, X60-X64, X85, and Y10-Y14. Rates shown are for the number of deaths per 100,000 population. Age-adjusted death rates were calculated using the direct method and the 2000 standard population.

† Drug overdose deaths, as defined, that have natural and semi-synthetic opioids (T40.2) as contributing causes.

§ Drug overdose deaths, as defined, that have methadone (T40.3) as a contributing cause.

¶ Categories of deaths are not exclusive as deaths may involve more than one drug. Summing of categories will result in greater than the total number of deaths in a year.

†† Analyses were limited to states meeting the following criteria: For states with very good to excellent reporting, ≥90% of drug overdose deaths mention at least one specific drug in 2014, with the change in percentage of drug overdose deaths mentioning at least one specific drug differing by < 10 percentage points between 2014 and 2015. States with good reporting had 80% – <90% of drug overdose deaths mention at least one specific drug in 2014, with the change in the percentage of drug overdose deaths mentioning at least one specific drug differing by <10 percentage points between 2014 and 2015. Rate comparisons between

States, Statistics & Death Certificates

Michigan

The state of Michigan has seen a rise in the number of overdose deaths over the past 15 years, with a record high in 2015, the most recent year of data available from the Michigan Department if Health and Human Services. Deaths related to opioid and heroin overdoses are a large part of the reason. In 1999, the state saw 62 opioid deaths and 37 heroin deaths. By 2014 there were **568 opioid deaths and 433 heroin deaths.**

Total all cause overdose deaths, including overdoses outside of heroin and opiates, climbed from 455 in 1999 to **1,745 in 2014**, according to information MDDHS extrapolated from Michigan death certificates.

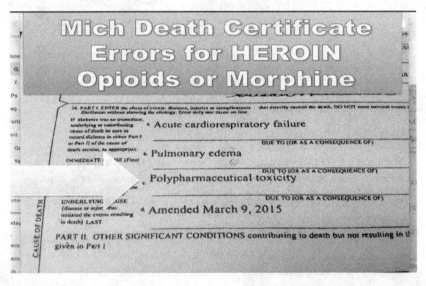

Death certificate data may be incomplete, fractured and inaccurate based on county variation, technology, and level of integration of medicolegal data.

We likely have more heroin deaths in America than we report.

Heroin deaths are often undercounted because of variations in state reporting procedures, and because heroin metabolizes into morphine very quickly in the body, making it difficult to determine the presence of heroin.

Many medical examiners are reluctant to characterize a death as heroin-related without the presence of *6-monoaceytlmorphine* (6-MAM), a metabolite unique to heroin deaths.

Further, there is no standardized system for reporting drug-related deaths in the United States. The manner of collecting and reporting death data varies with each medical examiner and coroner.

Opioid- and heroin-related deaths **(1,001)** make up more than half (57%) the total number for death certificate data in 2014.

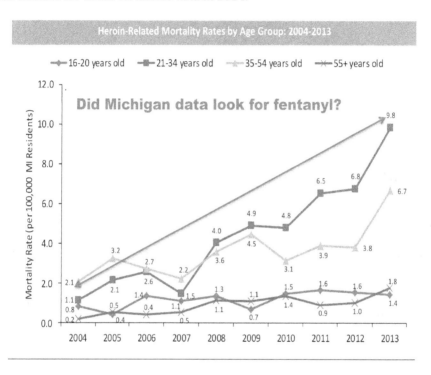

West Virginia

Fatal drug overdoses in West Virginia continued to rise last year and its overdose death rate still far outpaces any other state in the country.

A recent analysis by the West Virginia Health Statistics Center shows at least **818 people in the state died of drug overdoses** in 2016 — four times the number that occurred in 2001 and a nearly 13 percent increase over the 725 who died of overdoses in 2015.

About 86 percent of the deaths in 2016 involved at least one opioid.

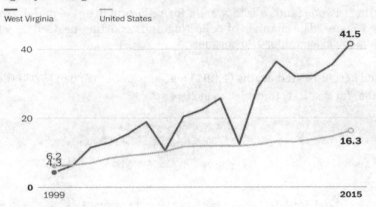

Drug overdose deaths surge in West Virginia

Age-adjusted drug overdose death rate, 1999 – 2015

West Virginia   United States

41.5

40

20

16.3

6.2
4.3

0

1999   2015

Sharp drops in West Virginia numbers in 2005 and 2009 may be due to data collection issues.

Source: CDC

WAPO.ST/WONKBLOG

Massachusetts

The number of opioid-related deaths in Massachusetts continues to climb, fueled by the use of fentanyl, a synthetic opiate that's often mixed with heroin, according to statistics released Monday by the state Department of Public Health.

There were 1,379 unintentional, opioid-related deaths in 2015, a seven percent increase from 2014.

As recently as 2012, there were fewer than 700 opioid-related deaths in the state.

State health officials said that for the first time the data included information about fentanyl and what they called its disturbing relationship to opioid-related deaths.

Officials said more than half of last year's confirmed opioid-related overdose deaths with a toxicology screen had a positive screen for fentanyl.

Ohio

There has been a 366% increase in Ohio drug overdose tests from 2000 to 2012. Unintentional drug overdoses have recently caused 3961 deaths in 2016.

Over this period of time, prescription drugs have been involved in most of the unintentional drug overdoses and have largely driven the rising deaths.

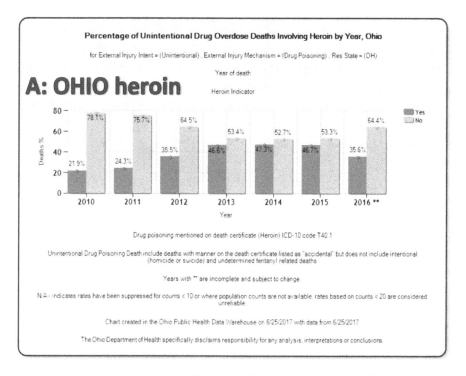

Percentage of Unintentional Drug Overdose Deaths Involving Heroin by Year, Ohio

for External Injury Intent = (Unintentional) , External Injury Mechanism = (Drug Poisoning) , Res State = (OH)

Year of death

A: OHIO heroin

Heroin Indicator

Drug poisoning mentioned on death certificate (Heroin) ICD-10 code T40.1

Unintentional Drug Poisoning Death include deaths with manner on the death certificate listed as "accidental" but does not include intentional (homicide or suicide) and undetermined fentanyl related deaths.

Years with ** are incomplete and subject to change.

N/A - indicates rates have been suppressed for counts < 10 or where population counts are not available. rates based on counts < 20 are considered unreliable.

Chart created in the Ohio Public Health Data Warehouse on 6/25/2017 with data from 6/25/2017

The Ohio Department of Health specifically disclaims responsibility for any analysis, interpretations or conclusions.

Data from 2012 reveal a significant shift in this trend, with an apparent leveling of prescription opioid related overdose doubts contrasted with a large increase in heroin related deaths. Heroin leading overdose deaths is new.

In 2013 the number of opioid overdose deaths caused by heroin exceeded the number of deaths involving prescription opioids.

The increasing flow of fentanyl is coming from the largely unregulated pharmaceutical industry in China. Some of the drug is exported directly to the United States, but it also pours in through Mexico and Canada.

Separately, results only from the Bureau of Criminal Investigation, a branch of Attorney General Mike DeWine's office, appear to back up the national report. The three BCI labs showed 2,396 positive tests for fentanyl in 2016, more than double the number in 2015 and 70 times the 34 fentanyl results in 2010. The drug samples are submitted to the lab for testing from law-enforcement agencies across the state as part of evidence gathering in criminal cases.

Forensic labs saw a drop in heroin test results, to 5,768 in 2016 from 6,832 in 2015, a nearly 16 percent decline. (see figure A: Ohio heroin)

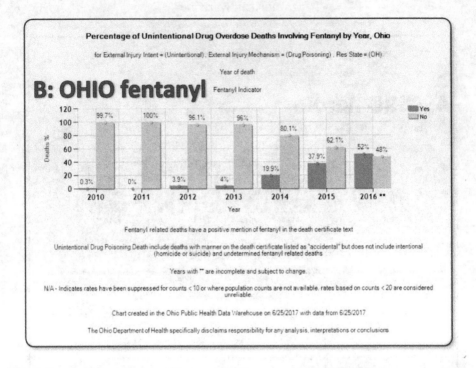

Ohio is at the epicenter of fentanyl abuse, as shown by laboratory tests from a number of agencies around the state of suspected illegal drugs confiscated by authorities. Ohio had 3,861 positive lab tests for fentanyl in 2015, more than four times the total in Pennsylvania, the next-highest state, with 897 results. (see figure: OHIO fentanyl)

Law-enforcement officers seized 368 pounds of illicit fentanyl in 2015, a significant amount considering that just 2 milligrams of the drug, which is equivalent to two grains of salt, can be fatal if inhaled or handled.

China is the primary source of fentanyl coming to the United States, from illegal manufacturing operations, the federal report said. The drug arrives in many forms, including counterfeit prescription pills, through parcels shipped in the mail and through shipping services, and smuggled across international borders. Fentanyl was responsible for 1,155 of the 3,050 drug overdose deaths in Ohio in 2015, the most recent year for which statistics are available. The fentanyl death toll more than doubled from 503 in 2014, according to the annual report from the Ohio Department of Health."

The narrative is simple. Heroin replaced prescription drug overdose deaths. Fentanyl is replacing or obscuring heroin overdose deaths. This will happen everywhere is America.

Akron, Ohio--EMS and police responded to a 911 call (6/2/17) at Gale and Colfax, to find an aparent heroin overdose that was reversed by EMS Narcan. This one year old baby boy is the youngest heroin overdose recorded by the Akron Children's Hospital. The second dose of Narcan was completed in the hospital. Pending toxicology will likely determine a heroin-fentanyl mix.

Ohio Drug Involvement by Year

Drug	2008	2010	2012	2014	2016
All opioids	735	979	1272	1,866	2,510
Rx opioids	546	694	680	672	799
heroin	233	338	697	1,194	**1,411**
fentanyl	6	5	75	503	**2,058**
All deaths	1,475	1,544	1,914	2,531	3,961
Crude rate/ 100k	12.8	13.4	16.6	18.8	20.4

Tennessee

In 2015, 1,451 people died of drug overdoses in Tennessee -- the highest annual number of overdose deaths in state history.

The data from the Tennessee Department of Health, brings the five-year total of overdose deaths, statewide, to 6,036 -- the same, the state said, as if every person on 40 mid-size jet airplanes died.

Almost 72 percent of those deaths, the state said, involved opioid drugs. About 30 percent combined opioid and benzodiazepine drugs, like Xanax.

Deaths caused by fentanyl, a powerful painkiller that rose in availability in East Tennessee over the past year, more than doubled: 174 deaths in 2015, up from 69 in 2014, the state said. Heroin associated deaths statewide increased to 205 in 2015, from 147 in 2015.

The Medical examiners throughout Florida have reported the spike in overdosed to us from heroin and the synthetic narcotic fentanyl. Michigan and Ohio are reporting the same forensic lab trends.

The trend is worse in South Florida. Palm Beach County was a horrific tragedy. More than 210 people died of heroin or related opioids in 2015.

492 heroin and opioid related deaths in Palm Beach County in 2015 and 2016

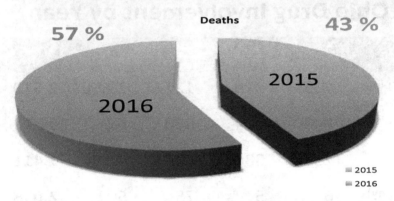

Palm Beach County related heroin and opioid deaths increased 14 % in 1 year.
http://www.mypalmbeachpost.com/wall/

Palm Beach County showed another deadly increase to 278 heroin or fentanyl related opioid deaths in 2016 and that accounted for approximately 40% of all deaths by drug intoxication.

Miami Dade County saw 100% jump in heroine deaths, and increases we're nearly 210% in Broward and 425% in Palm Beach counties.

Fentanyl deaths were up 310% in Miami-Dade and 100% in Broward.

Deaths from both drugs have skyrocketed nationwide.

The trends have continued through the end of 2016 into 2017.

South Florida users shifted to heroin (with fentanyl) after a crackdown on oxycodone.

Fentanyl, is 50 times stronger than heroin, is a prescription drug, but street fentanyls come from China and Mexico.

Pennsylvania

Out of a relatively small population of 1.85 million in West Virginia, 570 deaths from drug overdoses were recorded in that year. In Pennsylvania, with a much larger population, the number of overdose deaths was 2,426.

Prescription drugs accounted for more than half of the roughly 44,000 overdose deaths in the U.S. in 2013, the report found. Professionals started seeing increases in drug overdose deaths in the late '90s.

From 1997-2005 nationally, prescriptions increased 700 percent for OxyContin, 300 percent for hydrocodone and 1,000 percent for methadone, said Dr. Capretto, who was not involved in the report.

Though deaths from prescription drug overdoses peaked nationally around 2012, **heroin overdose** deaths have increased since then, leading to an overall uptick in deaths from drug overdoses.

Delaware

The cost of the pills skyrocketed as the supply dried up. A single 30-milligram Percocet can cost $30, according to the DEA for Pennsylvania and Delaware.

The heroin market responded with a drug that is more plentiful, purer and cheaper.

Twenty years ago, heroin was 17 percent pure and cost $10 a bag. Today, it's around 67 percent pure and can be purchased in Wilmington for as little as $3 a bag.

Even novice users from the suburbs know which parts of the city to visit to find a willing seller.

Rhode Island

Health officials say drug overdose deaths continue rising in Rhode Island, with a spike in fentanyl-related deaths last year.

The state health department said Wednesday that there were at least 326 drug overdose deaths in 2016 and 57 percent of those were fentanyl-related.
That's compared to 290 deaths in 2015, of which 47 percent were fentanyl-related.

Rhode Island deaths caused by prescription drugs has dropped over five years but deaths caused by illicit drug use are rising, with more overdoses caused by fentanyl.

The State Medical Examiners' data show that contrary to common assumptions, Rhode Island's drug overdose epidemic is not limited to younger adult males. While men accounted for twice as many accidental drug overdose deaths from 2009-2012, people ages 40 through 60 accounted for most of the drug overdose deaths overall.

"These data are of great concern to our department," said Craig Stenning, Director of BHDDH. "We are committed to continuing to develop effective prevention strategies and increasing access to treatment and recovery support services in an effort to help improve these statistics."

In Rhode Island, three key intervention strategies have been implemented over the last year in a concerted effort to address medication addiction, illicit prescription diversion, and accidental drug overdose deaths:

Naloxone, a medication that reverses an overdose from opioids (e.g. heroin, morphine, oxycodone) is now available without a prescription so that a layperson can help reverse a drug overdose of a friend or loved one.

Emergency medical professionals have used this safe and effective antidote for decades. In 2013, Walgreens became the first pharmacy chain to make Naloxone available without a prescription.

Good Samaritan Law. Callers to 911 now have immunity from prosecution if illicit drugs are involved in the emergency.

PDMP/PMP. HEALTH launched its Prescription Monitoring Program (PMP) in September of 2012. The PMP enables doctors, other prescribers, and pharmacists to monitor and protect patients from dangerous drug combinations and quantities, and helps reduce the amount of prescription drugs that can get into the hands of people without a prescription.

Colorado

Heroin deaths in 2016 grew by 23 percent, from 160 to 197.

Because the 2016 numbers are preliminary, they could still change before being finalized in the coming months. Health researchers aren't yet able to calculate death rates for 2016, which would show how the raw numbers compare to Colorado's rising population. Pro-Cannabis advocates are quick to point out that prescription opioid deaths are down in Colorado since the liberalization of cannabis policy.

The truth is that people struggling with substance use disorder have left oxycodone for heroin all over North America and Colorado is no different.

Show me that cannabis is reducing heroin use.

Opioid deaths have increased and this is reflected in heroin data.

None of these graphs are going in the right direction.

Death is not on holiday. The slopes are not slowing down. There is no attenuation.

By all measures heroin is out of control and naloxone is the only answer in every state. Prescription drug monitoring software does not stop deaths for heroin and naloxone does.

Ohio is proof that heroin is the big problem and while other states look to copy Ohio, nobody does the same thing after adopting the idea.

Task force members in every state wander away from heroin completeness.

Our lawmakers are late to the party and still looking at prescription overdoses.

California

3 million people abuse illegal drugs in California. Heroin is the second most common substance as a drug of choice on admission to public treatment facilities and agencies. Three out of ten fatal MVAs include and illegal drug.

Drug Abuse is the #1 cause of premature death in California.

Naloxone for Heroin-Fentanyl associated Mortality

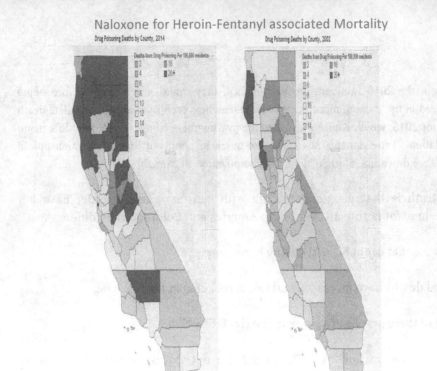

2014   2002

2014 versus 2002
drug poisoning deaths

Drug overdose deaths for 2014 are 4,521 and are most common and growing in far Northern California. These two maps show age-adjusted drug-poisoning death rates in California in 2002 and in 2014, according to the CDC.

Read more here: http://www.sacbee.com/site-services/databases/article56168810.html#storylink=cpy

National Heroin Threat Assessment (NHTA)

DEA's 2016 National Heroin Threat Assessment Summary outlines the growing public health crisis in the United States due to the use and abuse of heroin and other opioid drugs.

According to the report, the number of people reporting current heroin use tripled between 2007 and 2014, while the number of deaths involving the drug tripled between 2010 and 2014.

The number of deaths due to synthetic opioids such as fentanyl rose 79% from 2013 to 2014. The report includes for the first time information on fentanyl disguised as prescription drugs, something reportedly behind the deaths of 19 people in Florida and California in the first quarter of this year.

"We tend to overuse words such as 'unprecedented' and 'horrific,' but the death and destruction connected to heroin and opioids is indeed unprecedented and horrific," said DEA Acting Administrator Chuck Rosenberg.

Many users of controlled prescription drugs (CPDs) become addicted to opioid medications originally prescribed for valid medical purposes.

The report noted that heroin today is higher in purity, less expensive, and may be easier to obtain than illegal CPDs.

New to this year's summary is information on a recent phenomenon—fentanyl disguised as prescription pills—something allegedly responsible for the death of 19 people in Florida and California during the first quarter of 2016.

Motivated by enormous profit potential, traffickers are exploiting high consumer demand for illicit prescription painkillers, tranquilizers, and sedatives by producing inexpensive counterfeits containing fentanyl that can be sold on the street.

The number of users, treatment admissions, overdose deaths, and seizures from traffickers all increased over those reported in last year's summary. In addition, heroin was the greatest drug threat reported by 45 percent (up from 38% last year and 7% in 2007) of state, local, and tribal law enforcement agencies responding to the 2016 National Drug Threat Survey, an annual survey of a representative national sample of 2,761 agencies.

And while the heroin threat is particularly high in the Northeast, Mid-Atlantic, and Midwest areas of the United States, law enforcement agencies in cities across the country report seizing larger than usual quantities of heroin.

National Seizure System data show an 80 percent increase in heroin seizures in the past five years, from 3,733 kilograms in 2011 to 6,722 kilograms in 2015.

(U) Despite comprising a smaller user population, there were more treatment admissions to publicly funded facilities for heroin than for any other drug. (See Chart 9.)

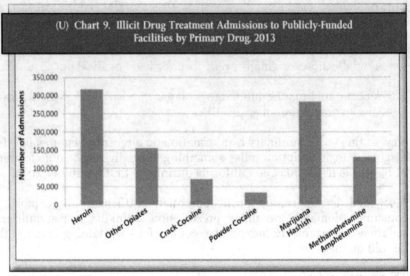

(U) Chart 9. Illicit Drug Treatment Admissions to Publicly-Funded Facilities by Primary Drug, 2013

Source: Treatment Episode Data Set

DEA News Release (06/27/16)

https://www.dea.gov/divisions/hq/2016/hq062716.shtml

Heroin Short-Term Effects:

Euphoria

Warm flushing of skin

Dry mouth

Heavy feeling in the hands and feet

Clouded thinking

Alternate wakeful and drowsy states

Itching

Nausea

Vomiting

Slowed breathing and heart rate

Heroin Long-Term Effects:

Collapsed Veins

Abscesses (swollen tissue with pus)

Infection of the lining and valves in the heart

Constipation and stomach cramps

Liver or kidney disease

Pneumonia

Medications to Treat Heroin Addiction:

Methadone

Buprenorphine

Naltrexone (oral short- and I.M. XR long-acting forms)
And Naloxone I.V., S.C., I.M., and I.N. for overdose

Behavioral Therapies:

Contingency management, or motivational incentives

12-Step facilitation therapy

Suppliers put Fentanyl and fentanyl structures in the heroin. **Fentanyl is driving opioid overdose deaths higher:**

fentanyl

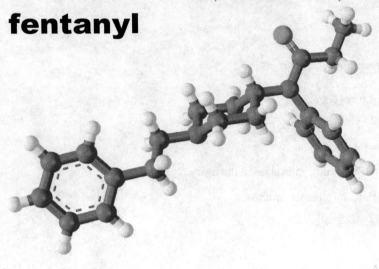

In Kent County from 2010 to 2015 heroin related deaths increased from 13% to 30% and Bay County saw a similar increase, while deaths from methadone decreased over the same time period.

Over the last three years in particular, Fentanyl has emerged as a significant factor driving the increase in opioid overdose deaths. CDC issued fentanyl reports in June 2013 and August 2013 and a Health Alert in October 2015.[i] In March 2015, Drug Enforcement Agency (DEA) issued a nationwide Alert on Fentanyl as a Threat to Health and Public Safety.

DEA Administrator Michele M. Leonhart commented "Drug incidents and overdoses related to fentanyl are occurring at an alarming rate throughout the United States and represent a significant threat to public health and safety".[ii]

As we highlight below, fentanyl is implicated in high proportions (14% to 66%) of opioid overdose deaths in some states, up from mid-single digits just a new years ago.

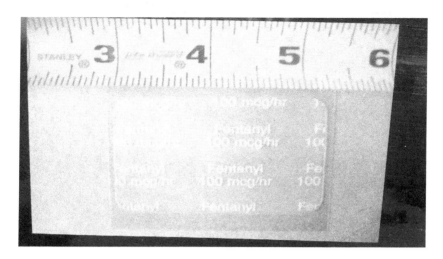

he two fentanyls include both prescription fentanyl and illicitly manufactured fentanyl. Also called Non-Prescription Fentanyl (NPF).

Prescription fentanyl's respiratory depressive effects peak in 5-15 minutes and, depending on dose, these effects may last for many hours.[iii]

While fentanyl overdoses can be reversed with naloxone, because of fentanyl's potency, rapid onset and long lasting respiratory depressive effects, the window of intervention may be narrower and a higher dose of naloxone may be needed.

As CDC states in its October 2015 Health Alert "Multiple doses of naloxone may need to be administered per overdose event because of fentanyl's increased potency relative to other opioids"[iv]

According to the 2015 released data from the U.S. Centers for Disease Control and Prevention (CDC), 5,500 people died of synthetic opioid overdoses in 2014, most of them related to fentanyl. That's an 80% increase over the numbers reported in 2013.

The Drug Enforcement Administration issued a national alert stating that "drug incidents and overdoses related to fentanyl are occurring at an alarming rate." In 2013, the DEA made 942 fentanyl seizures; in 2014, it made 3,344.

CDC data from 2016 released on 2015 fentanyl deaths show greater than 9,000 overdosed involved fentanyl.

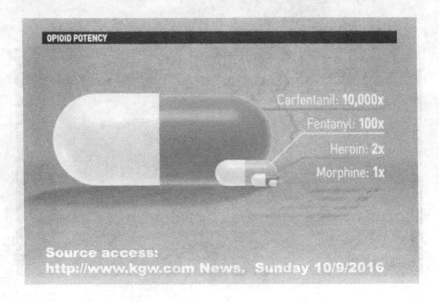

Why are the drug suppliers now using fentanyl family products? In the past model they were cutting heroin with junk to stretch it for making more profit.

The future is a shift to cut heroin with chemicals to brand it as more potent. This is a change in the heroin supply chain model. Someday they may just supply fentanyl, which has proven to be more deadly.

Naloxone Assessment: Hiding in Egypt, When Herod Was King.

The opioid overdose epidemic worsened further in 2015 claiming approximately 33,000 lives according to Centers for Diseases Control and Prevention (CDC). Opioid overdose is characterized by life-threatening respiratory and central nervous system (CNS) depression that, if not immediately treated, may lead to significant morbidity and mortality due to irreversible hypoxic injury.

Table 1. Number of drug poisoning deaths by category, United States, 2011-2014

	2011	2012	2013	2014 (% Change 2013-2014)	% Change 2012-2013	% Change 2011-2013	% Change 2011-2014	2015 MMWR DATA
All drug Total deaths	41,340	41,502	43,982	47,055 (+6.5%)	6.00	6.40	13.8	52,404 (+12%)
Heroin deaths	4,397	5,925	8,257	10,574 (+26.0)	39.40	87.80	140.48	12,990 (+23%)
Rx opioid deaths	16,917	16,007	16,235	18,073 (+11.3)	1.40	-4.00	6.83	20,101 (+12%)

Source: Modified Center for Disease Control and Prevention, (CDC Wonder) Available at http://www.cdc.gov/. All opioid deaths 33,091 and 9,000 fentanyl (>70%)

12,990 – heroin deaths

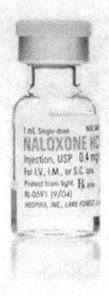

Naloxone Assessment

Naloxone is an effective treatment for opioid overdose if a sufficient dose is administered in time.

Consequently, a key element of the consensus comprehensive policy response to the epidemic is to expand naloxone access to lay persons in non-healthcare settings where the vast majority of opioid overdose related deaths happen.[v]

The Food and Drug Administration (FDA) has supported this policy by fast tracking and approving, under priority review, two new formulations of naloxone (Evzio® (naloxone hydrochloride auto-injector) and Narcan® (naloxone hydrochloride) Nasal Spray).

Future potential naloxone formulations have been granted fast track status by FDA. Oral Naloxone has not been developed to be significantly available through the stomach for rapid applications. It is injected somewhere in the body or sprayed up the nose.

Large doses of oral naloxone have been shown to be efficacious in reversing opioid-induced constipation. However, they often cause the unwanted side effect of *analgesia reversal*. This is the desired effect in heroin overdose reversal.

You must appreciate heroin next to naloxone. Naloxone is not psychoactive and binds to the brain in a way that pushes heroin out of the brain. How does Naloxone work?

Naloxone looks like heroin and may share 85-90 % of the 3-D structural chemistry.

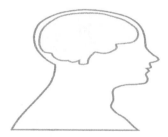

When Naloxone is administered it pushes heroin off the brain.

Timely administration of a sufficient naloxone dose by a trained layperson or emergency medical services responder can reverse fentanyl overdose.

Although bystanders were frequently present in the general location of overdose death, timely bystander naloxone administration did not occur because bystanders did not have naloxone, were spatially separated or impaired by substance use, or failed to recognize overdose symptoms.

Findings indicate that persons using fentanyl have an increased chance of surviving an overdose if directly observed by someone trained and equipped with sufficient doses of naloxone.

The overdose is reversed when enough heroin is pushed off the brain by naloxone which looks like heroin. People start breathing again.

A) **Naloxone above. B) Heroin below.**

B)

Wrongly, Physicians, Lawyers, and legislative consultants have argued that if you reverse people they will use again.

Yes.

Yes they will. But they are not dead.

THE ARGUMENT

- THE ARGUMENT: if you reverse OD with naloxone you allow people to use I.V. drugs again is **fatally** flawed.
- **Reversing overdose stops death.**
- You mix and confound arguments about two discreet events.
- These arguments do not belong mixed.
- Dead people cannot start treatment.

Public health centered naloxone approaches with federal, state and local authorities can effectively reduce overdose risk and fatality rates.

Together, improved gathering and timely dissemination of critical drug-related information, expansion of access to naloxone, and provision of basic legal protections for good Samaritans or medical personnel are seminal.

An intellectually honest and a genuine exploration of novel strategies, can prevent fatal overdoses.

The Michigan Standing Order created by PA 383 is a cornerstone to a new testament's naloxone policy. One master medical executive prescription executed as a standing order for all retail pharmacies is a sweet victory. Pharmacists are the new "Gatekeepers" demons from the heroin overdose epidemic that has swept through Pennsylvania, Ohio, Michigan, Indiana and America these last 3-4 years.

This is a victory for families that have family members struggling with addiction. There is always a cost. What is the cost? The cost was the lack of engagement and understanding by primary care physicians and regional healthcare systems. 240 hospitals in Michigan and community naloxone prescribing is absent in 97% of them. 40,000 physicians in Michigan and community naloxone prescribing is absent in 99.8% of them. The majority of Michigan doctors fail to grasp the seriousness of the overdose deaths and the tools to stop the dying.

Healthcare systems are promoting a community flu shot the CDC rates at 48 % effective. Healthcare systems ignore community naloxone that is 99.99 % effective.

41

The CDC estimates 200,000 hospitalizations and **36,000 deaths from flu**. The CDC recorded **33,000 opioid overdose deaths** in its last report.

Kochanek, et al (2011) illustrates 32 ED admissions for each death; that is **1,056,000** visits to ED for overdose from abuse and misuse of opioids in MI. This is before heroin use tripled in America.

Who is at highest risk to overdose?

One predictor of increased likelihood to overdose was having a previous history of overdose. When I queried 18 drug court participants on fear of overdose the surprizing answer was zero percent feared overdose and 100 % feared withdrawal. Can you predict overdose risk and stratify that risk in pain or addiction patients?

Who is at risk for an overdose?

- people with opioid dependence, in particular those with reduced tolerance (following detoxification, release from incarceration, cessation of treatment)
- people who inject opioids
- people who use prescription opioids, in particular those on higher doses
- people who use opioids in combination with other sedating substances
- opioid users with other significant medical conditions (HIV, liver or lung disease, depression)
- **household members of people in possession of strong opioids** VERY SMALL **CHILDREN**

Enter the retail pharmacist and the retail pharmacy; life saving medication and the education to use it in the community with no appointment needed.

As the opioid epidemic evolves, we must also evolve how we approach the use and access of naloxone. First responders and EMTs are no longer the only ones facing this problem head on, and cannot be the only people equipped with naloxone and plenty of it.

Now, addiction medicine and public health doctors, harm reduction groups, friends, treatment centers, law enforcement, family and community members are finding themselves at the frontlines of this epidemic and able to impact these emergency situations in unparalleled ways.

Therefore, We must make a promise to get naloxone into the homes and hands of the general public in order to prevent these overdose-related deaths from even occurring and slowing this public health crisis. It is the only way to give Americans in the throes of addiction a second chance at life.

That is why, as doctors, educators and pain specialists, it has been our mission to not only carefully slow the prescribing and proliferation of non-medical opioid drugs, but to spread the knowledge of and access to this potentially life-saving medication in the communities that need it most.

Today, there are FDA-approved naloxone products intended for community use and made with the non-medically trained person in mind, including mothers, brothers or caregivers.

Thankfully, there have been significant breakthroughs in the battle against our nation's opioid epidemic through increased access to naloxone.

Currently, 37 states have issued standing orders, which permits pharmacies to dispense naloxone without a physician's prescription, meaning anyone in these 37 states can walk into a CVS, Rite-Aid, Walgreens, Target, Wal-Mart or independent pharmacy and request an easy-to-use, pharmacy supported naloxone without a prescription.

WEYI ch-25 NBC/ch-66 FOX called all four hospitals in the Midland Bay Saginaw (MBS) tri-county area the day of the Heroin Summit (03/16/2017) at the Grace A. Dow Memorial Library in Midland. St. Mary's Ascension Health never replied.

McLaren, MidMichigan and Covenant returned calls but all admitted they had no addiction medicine department and no addiction specialists on staff to deal with the treatment needed. Paralysis has an antidote. Where hospitals are pondering, retail pharmacies will be kinetic and stand in the gap. Ezekial 22:30

In recent months, large pharmacy retailers have begun rolling out programs across the nation to provide naloxone to lay persons without a patient specific prescription, under various state naloxone prescribing laws, protocols or local collaborative practice agreements, which is referred to as, Standing Order Access, in this State of the State report.

In 37 states, you can purchase naloxone from a pharmacist directly without getting a prescription.

Improvised Nasal Naloxone

There is widespread non-FDA approved use of pre-filled vial(s) of naloxone 2mg/2ml for injection and non-FDA approved instructions for assembly immediately prior to administration and dose titration.

The use of Improvised Nasal Naloxone looks set to be expanded to laypersons as pharmacy retailers implement Standing Order naloxone access.

In the context of the availability of new FDA approved naloxone formulations, the continued and expanded use of Improvised Nasal Naloxone raises the following serious concerns.

Put simply, what little published data exist about Improvised Nasal Naloxone suggest it is complex to administer (resulting in a high error rate) and delivers less naloxone more slowly than the lowest FDA approved dose. This dosing concern comes just as more potent opioids that need stronger naloxone doses drive the overdose death rate ever higher. Other experts in the overdose arena publicly shared similar concerns include:

Dr John Strang of the National Addiction Centre, Institute of Psychiatry, Psychology and Neuroscience, King's College London, London, UK who published a debate paper in Addiction journal titled "Clinical provision of improvised nasal naloxone without experimental testing and without regulatory approval: imaginative shortcut or dangerous bypass of essential safety procedures? He concludes that "… clinicians should prescribe take-home naloxone only as one of its licensed formulations, since it remains uncertain how adequately and reliably the improvised nasal spray is absorbed".[vi]

Dr. Phil Skolnick, of the National Institutes on Drug Abuse in a recent media report in the International Business Times said "he can't imagine why physicians would prescribe or recommend the old nasally administered version, now that Narcan nasal spray is available. "For me, it would be unethical to use anything else," he says."[vii]

Dr. Sharon Hertz of Director, Division of Anesthesia, Analgesia, and Addiction Products, Office of New Drugs, Center for Drug Evaluation and Research, FDA in a MedPage article commented "Though appropriate for medical settings where patients' breathing and blood pressure can be supported, the incremental administration of smaller doses of naloxone to minimize withdrawal symptoms takes more time and medical expertise than may be available in an emergency."[viii]

Separately Dr Hertz commented in the Summary Review for Regulatory Action of Narcan Nasal Spray "There is evidence that the off-label use of naloxone by the intranasal route has been effective in reversing opioid overdose in many cases.

However, there are no data that specifically quantitate the success rate, leaving the question of whether there are situations that could have benefited from a higher dose of naloxone. Unpublished pharmacokinetic data suggest that naloxone levels following off-label use by the intranasal route are lower than by the approved routes of administration.".[ix]

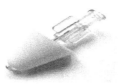

MAD

Dr Tim Wolfe, inventor of the Mucosal Atomizer Device (MAD) used in the Improvised Nasal Naloxone and editor of intranasasl.net stated "Even though I invented the MAD nasal, began the research on nasal naloxone in the 1990s and have used this therapy for 18 years (so have a bit of a historical bent towards the original method of delivery), it seems pretty apparent to me that this new product is probably a better method for delivery of nasal naloxone than the way we have posted here on this website for the last 7 years.

The new formulation is more appropriately concentrated, it has a pre-attached atomizer and because of the recent price increased in generic naloxone (single supplier cranked the price last year) this new formulation is not only better formulated, it's also less expensive."[x]

Improvised Nasal Naloxone vs FDA approved Narcan

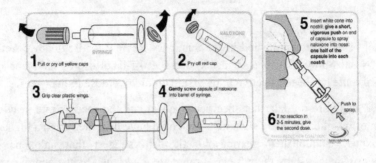

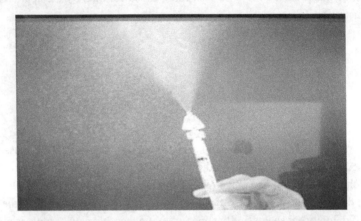

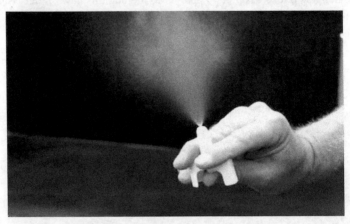

Naloxone Formulations-Pharmacokinetics

Route	Dose	C_{max} (pg/mL)	T_{max} (hr)	AUC1-hr (hr-pg/mL)	$t_{1/2}$ (hr)	Ref
IV	0.036 mg/kg	26270 ± 11890*	0.05	12730 ± 2550*	NR	1
IN	20 mg Crushed Powder	20180 ± 5710*	0.28	29830 ± 12470*	NR	1
IN	4 mg (NARCAN) *	4830 (43.1%)	0.5	7980 (37.3%)	2.08 (29.8%)	2
IM	2 mg (Syringe)	4160 (43.9%)	0.25	8088 (13.5%)	1.47 (24.2%)	3
IN	2 mg (Off label kit)	1163 (47.6%)	0.25	1411 (36.7%)	1.44 (17.2%)	3
IM/SC	0.4 mg (EVZIO) *	1100 (52.4%)	0.25	1880 (24.7%)	1.22 (28.2%)	4
IM/SC	0.4 mg (Syringe)	857 (53.2%)	0.33	1910 (27.5%)	1.32 (22%)	4
IN	2 mg+ oxy (Off label kit)	871 (48.9%)	0.33	1077 (36.3%)	1.48 (20.7%)	3

* Data presented as mean ± SD. Other data presented as geometric mean (gCV%); Ref # 3 oxy is decongestant oxymetazoline.

Data generated by third parties indicate the bioavailability of Improvised Nasal Naloxone may be so low that less naloxone is delivered than the lowest approved dose of naloxone administered by intramuscular injection. Third party sources include

Dowling et al. 2008 studied the comparative bioavailability of intranasal naloxone and injectable naloxone in 6 healthy volunteers and concluded the relative bioavailability of nasal naloxone was 4%.[xi]

Strang et al. 2015 estimated the bioavailability of Improvised Nasal Naloxone to be approximately 10% - based on an assumed 40% bioavailability and a nasal cavity volume capacity of 0.25ml per nostril. Each vial of Improvised Nasal Naloxone contains 2ml of liquid. They concluded that the Improvised Nasal Naloxone would deliver oxone dose "equivalent to only half the lower recommended injectable dose. The remainder would be lost as nasal drip or as post-nasal drip (and inactivaton)." [xii]

Data from a pilot PK study in 12 subjects conducted by AntiOp, Inc. (published in a patent application)[xiii] characterized the PK of Improvised Nasal Naloxone, naloxone administered by injection and a proposed nasal naloxone spray from Indivior plc. These published data indicate Improvised Nasal Naloxone delivers half of the lowest FDA approved intravenous dose of naloxone. (Chart 1).

In addition, in the same study, Improvised Nasal Naloxone was shown to deliver less naloxone more slowly than the proposed nasal naloxone spray from Indivior plc – a product which received a complete response letter from FDA according to Indivior because "...the early stage uptake of naloxone nasal spray did not fully meet the FDA's threshold as determined by the reference product (0.4 mg naloxone by intramuscular injection)".[xiv]

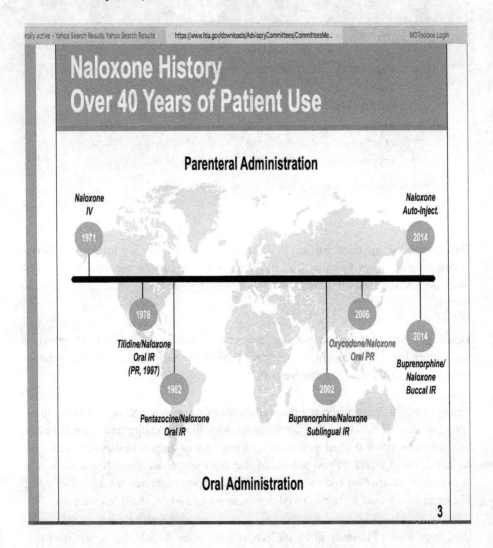

Figure 1. Mean Naloxone Plasma Concentration of Improvised Nasal Naloxone 2mg/2ml (2mg Amph) and naloxone 0.4mg delivered by intravenous injection (0.4mg IV) in 1st hour post dose.

Figure 2. Mean Naloxone Plasma Concentration of Improvised Nasal Naloxone 2mg/2ml (2mg Amph) and naloxone 2mg delivered by intranasal spray not approved by FDA (Indivior) in 1st hour post dose

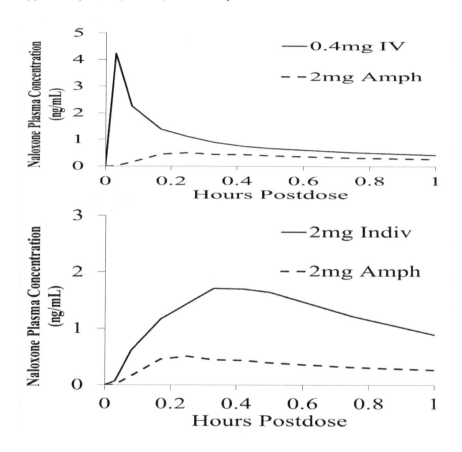

Source: *US Patent 9,192,570;*

WO 2015/095644 AntiOp, Inc.

From the IrishTimes.com:

Indivior's nasal spray rejected by FDA

Sprays contain naloxone, a drug that has been used to treat opioid overdose

Wed, Nov 25, 2015, 21:54

"Indivior said on Tuesday that the US Food and Drug Administration rejected its nasal spray for the emergency treatment of opioid overdose. The company is reviewing the health regulator's response.

These sprays contain naloxone, a drug that has been used to treat opioid overdose for nearly 45 years in injectable forms.

Last week, the FDA approved the first-ever nasal spray formulation of the drug made by Adapt Pharma Ltd, the Dublin-based start-up of entrepreneur Seamus Mulligan. Adapt expects to start marketing its product, Narcan, in January.

The FDA has been speeding up its review of new formulations of nalaxone to combat rising opioid abuse."

Assembly and titration

The improvised instructions for assembly and administration of Improvised Nasal Naloxone include four assembly and two titration steps for each vial. It is unknown whether lay persons can successfully assemble and titrate the Improvised Nasal Naloxone or the time required to do so. Published data (Edwards et al, Pain and Therapy 2015) report significant challenges with administration. (See below) As the Improvised Nasal Naloxone transitions to Behind the Counter availability, the lack of understanding of the complexity of administration and titration for laypersons in an emergency situation is of great concern.

Pain and Therapy 2015, Edwards et al published results of a study in 42 subjects comparing the usability of a naloxone auto-injector device and Improvised Nasal Naloxone in the administration of naloxone during a simulated opioid overdose emergency. In the study, absent device training, no participant successfully administered a simulated naloxone dose of Improvised Nasal Naloxone, after device training only 57% did so correctly. The time involved in administering the Improvised Nasal Naloxone product was also significant at an average of 6 minutes before training and over 2 minutes after training.[xv]

While titration for a medically trained person, in a hospital setting with a known opioid being antagonized may be preferable, this dosing appears a lot more challenging for non-medically trained lay persons, in non-healthcare settings when the opioid been antagonized in unlikely to be known.

Dr. Sharon Hertz of Director, Division of Anesthesia, Analgesia, and Addiction Products, Office of New Drugs, Center for Drug Evaluation and Research, FDA, commented in the Summary Review for Regulatory Action of Narcan Nasal Spray that "The benefit of using an incremental approach [to dosing] is that it may be possible to avoid precipitating an acute withdrawal syndrome in an opioid-tolerant patient, although this risk is outweighed if it means lessening the likelihood of reversing the overdose and re-establishing spontaneous reparations capable of providing adequate ventilation and oxygenation." [xvi]

Consistently adequate dose

The Improvised Nasal Naloxone may deliver a dose of naloxone that is not consistently adequate to reverse opioid overdoses in the context of the rapid rise of more potent fentanyl and illicitly manufactured fentanyl (NPF) which is a major driver of the growth in the overdose epidemic.[xvii] As Dr. Janet Woodcock, director of the FDA's Center for Drug Evaluation and Research stated in the FDA press release announcing the approval of Narcan Nasal Sprat "We heard the public call for this new route of administration, and we are happy to have been able to move so quickly on a product we are confident will deliver consistently adequate levels of the medication – a critical attribute for this emergency life-saving drug," said

Following an outbreak of deaths involving fentanyl in Rhode Island in 2013, CDC issued an advisory stating "….larger doses of naloxone may be required to reverse the opioid induced respiratory depression because of the higher potency of fentanyl and acetyl fentanyl compared to heroin.

CDC advises that emergency departments and emergency medical services ensure that they have adequate naloxone available, as some agencies have run out of naloxone in the face of increased numbers of overdoses and administering higher doses of naloxone in a short period of time."[xviii]

Since 2013, the number of opioid overdose deaths has soared and CDC issued a Health Advisory October 2015 stating "While NPF-related overdoses can be reversed with naloxone, a higher dose or multiple number of doses per overdose event may be required to revive a patient due to the high potency of NPF".[xix]

In the winter of 2017, Saginaw, Michigan K-9 unit called me just after midnight one morning and reported they delivered 8 rounds of Improvised Nasal Naloxone to a male on scene and it completely depleted all of the officer's naloxone that I had supplied.

Within 12 hours, I met them for late breakfast and delivered another 100 vials of naloxone. The lab testing at E.D. St. Mary's is not capable of separating out morphine, heroin or fentanyl family compounds. It is highly likely he did not have organic generic garden variety heroin.

The fentanyl family addition to heroin has been a game changer to the naloxone reversal treatments and strategy all across America.

While additional doses may be available in healthcare settings, there can be no assurance that first responders in the field or laypersons equipped with Improvised Nasal Naloxone will be able to administer an adequate dose.

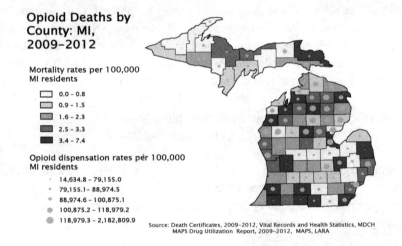

Source: Death Certificates, 2009–2012, Vital Records and Health Statistics, MDCH
MAPS Drug Utilization Report, 2009–2012, MAPS, LARA

A dynamic epidemic

The examples below serve to highlight how prevalent fentanyl has become in opioid overdose deaths, and the need for stronger doses of naloxone.

- In Ohio fentanyl-related unintentional drug overdose deaths increased from 84 in 2013, involving fewer than 4 percent of such deaths, to 502 in 2014, involving 20.2 percent of such deaths.[xx]

- In Maryland fentanyl-related unintentional drug overdose deaths increased from 58 in 2013 to 185 in 2014, representing 17% of opioid overdose related deaths.[xxi]

- Research indicate that fentanyl was implicated in the deaths of 37% of opioid overdoses in Massachusetts in the first half of 2014.[xxii]

- In Florida, 397 fatal overdoses were attributed to fentanyl in 2014, up from 185 in 2013.[xxiii]

- In Rhode Island, 50% of overdose deaths in 2015 involved fentanyl, up from 37% in 2014, and far higher than prior years, where less than 5% of deaths involved fentanyl.[xxiv]

- In Maine the Attorney General reports that in the first half of 2015, fentanyl was implicated in 25% of opioid overdose deaths.[xxv]

- In New Hampshire according to a New Hampshire Department of Health and Human Services fentanyl has been implicated in 2/3rd of the overdose deaths in the first 8 months of 2015.[xxvi]

- In Pennsylvania fentanyl was implicated in 14% of opioid overdose deaths in 2014.[xxvii]

- In Connecticut fentanyl is implicated in 23% of opioid overdose related deaths in the nine months ended September 2015.[xxviii]

- In Delaware fentanyl is implicated in 31 deaths in the first nine months of 2015 versus 11 for all of 2014. Based on an extrapolation of reported overdoses through July 2015 this indicates fentanyl is implicate din approximately 22% of overdose deaths.[xxix]

- In Vermont fentanyl is implicated in 32% of opioid overdose deaths in 2014.[xxx]

- In Virginia fentanyl is implicated in 28% of opioid overdose deaths in 2014.[xxxi]

Specific recent cases of more potent opioids requiring larger doses of naloxone include:

In an October 2015 outbreak in Chicago where there were 74 overdoses in 72 hours, related to heroin and fentanyl, Diane Hincks, a registered nurse and emergency room director at Mount Sinai on the West Side commenting on those overdosing stated "They're taking double and triple the doses [of naloxone hydrochloride] in order to bring them out of their stupor,"[xxxii]

In Ocean County, New Jersey in response to the outbreak of fentanyl related overdoses the police force started carrying double doses of Improvised Nasal Naloxone.[xxxiii]

In Erie County, New York 23 people died in February 2016 as a result of overdose on what is believed to be heroin laced with fentanyl. For those saved it took repeated doses of naloxone to reverse the opioid overdose.[xxxiv]

New FDA approved alternative treatments

FDA approved Evzio® (naloxone hydrochloride auto-injector) in 2014. Each carton includes a training device and 2 auto-injectors – each unit delivers 2 mg naloxone hydrochloride intramuscularly via an auto-injector device. The product is ready-to-use and can be used by non-medically trained personnel. The Wholesaler Acquisition Cost (WAC) is $3,500 for each package containing two devices and a training device.

FDA approved Narcan® (naloxone hydrochloride) Nasal Spray 4mg in November 2015. Each carton contains two devices, each unit contains 4mg naloxone concentrated in a single 0.1ml spray. In a pivotal pharmacokinetic study the dose normalized relative bioavailability of a single 4mg dose of Narcan Nasal Spray compared to 0.4mg administered by intramuscular injection was 46.7%. Narcan is also now a 2 mg nasal spray. The product is ready-to-use and needle free and can be used by non-medically trained personnel. Narcan Nasal Spray can be accessed at a discounted Public Interest Price of $37.50 per dose ($75 per carton of two devices) by first responders, state and local purchasers and non-for-profits. The WAC is $125 per carton containing 2 devices (equivalent of $62.50 per device). The product also has broad insurance coverage in approximately 82% of covered lives.

Conclusion

Retail pharmacists have a chance to replace physicians as a source of a life saving medication and disease education in the heroin overdose epidemic. Pharmacist have better hours, access and placement logistics. Is this fatal flaw in naloxone uptake squarely on the backs of physicians or the military-industrial-hospital-physician complex? Why would the healthcare matrix want to screen, question and treat substance use disorder with any naloxone?

Because it is socially responsible.

There are not enough credentialed addiction treatment providers in America.

350,000,000 people in America and 3,500 active addiction specialists. That is one addiction specialist for every 100,000 people.

There are not enough addiction treatment facilities in America.

The state of Michigan (like others) has to reconstruct pathways to care and change to retail pharmacists because of poor uptake in primary care physicians.

The administration of Improvised Nasal Naloxone has unquestionably saved many lives. Especially New York City unintentional drug poisoning deaths from 2005-10.

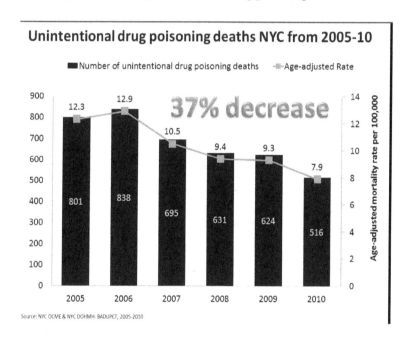

However, the opioid overdose epidemic is dynamic and more potent opioids are now driving death rates higher. Additionally, FDA has now approved new formulation(s) of naloxone that can be administered by laypersons in non-healthcare settings and deliver a consistently adequate dose.

Communities, retailers and state and local governmental agencies are rapidly scaling-up expanded naloxone access as a key element of the consensus policy response to the epidemic. To successfully implement this policy it is critical that naloxone product(s) underpinning this policy have been reviewed and approved by FDA and are appropriate for a dynamic epidemic and use by lay persons in community settings.

In the context of the concerns outlined in this document and the availability of new FDA approved naloxone formulation options we urge pharmacy retailers to balance the distribution of the Improvised Nasal Naloxone, as there are serious concerns about whether it is fit for purpose, and train pharmacists on FDA approved formulations.

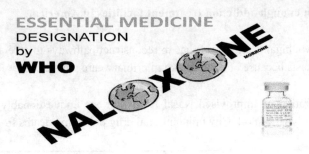

Naloxone is the equalizer:

In the end, it is the retail pharmacists entering an epidemic with naloxone to reduce the carnage of our youth. The last tragedy that records the senseless death of our children was "hiding in Egypt, when Herod was king."

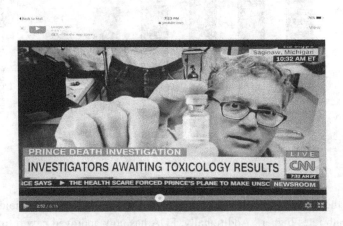

American Medical Association (AMA)

Naloxone is a lifesaving medication, introduced more than 40 years ago. A health care provider, family member or friend can administer it to someone experiencing an opioid overdose. It blocks the opioid's effects, helps restore breathing and prevents death.

The AMA encourages states to make Naloxone more available and provides information for physicians to prescribe Naloxone.

Co-prescribing Naloxone With Opioids
Physicians are encouraged to co-prescribe Naloxone to patients or prescribe it for a family member or close friend when clinically appropriate.

Factors to consider when determining whether to co-prescribe Naloxone:

the patient is on a high opioid dose

the patient has a concomitant benzodiazepine, sedative hypnotic prescription

the patient has a history of substance use disorder or in treatment.

the patient has an underlying mental condition that might make him or her more susceptible to overdose.

the patient has a medical condition, such as a respiratory disease or other co-morbidities, which might make him or her susceptible to opioid toxicity, respiratory distress or overdose.

the patient has young children or teens in the home.

the patient might be in a position to aid someone.

Obama & HHS/ASPE 2015 SUD policy

Opioid overdose related death and hospital visits have reached alarming levels

Naloxone to play a role in HHS opioid overdose initiative[1]

- **Opioid Prescribing Practices** to reduce opioid use disorders and overdose
- Expanded use and distribution of **Naloxone**
- Expansion of **Medication-assisted Treatment (MAT)** to reduce opioid use disorders and overdose

Detailing_Provider_final- booklet.pdf (page 4 of 1)

HHS/ASPE policy has not changed for SUD between President Obama and President Trump.

Both administrations have recognized the need to help those struggling with addiction.

The greatest variance comes from points presented at the 2015 President Obama conclave of governors at the White House.

Each state assembled their governor's task force and submitted this process to their political appointees. We see the pound of flesh principal introduced by Shakspear.

What had been originally taught as President Obama's 3 point plan has been translated in each state. Obviously 22 members of a state task force must produce a 22 point plan.

The message from Washington is the same. It is more likely that the state of politics in each state has not translated from Washington DC. Some states took the Obama message and created opioid commissions as fronts for witch-hunts to put doctors in jail instead of expand naloxone programs.

Sometimes the Obama plan is still recognizable in the state plan and sometimes it is not. The Obama message was crystal clear. The Obama message was the 3 points repeated over and over by:

ONDCP director Michael Botticelli

HHS secretary Sylvia Burwell

ASPE assistant secretary Richard Frank

How do we stop people dying?

• Naloxone Co-prescription and 3rd party prescribing to high risk groups

• Stop prescriptions of opioids to people with inappropriate risk benefit ratios

• Expand MAT treatment

2015 PCSS-O

Naloxone must be the foundation of the plan. Naloxone must be the heart of any plan. Naloxone must be the litmus test of all plans. Naloxone advocates must be the drivers of policy and intellectual honesty.

Naloxone answers the question that you end up with about "What do I do about prescription overdose deaths or heroin overdose deaths?"

Naloxone compensates for not enough addiction providers. Naloxone is more important than prescription drug monitoring software.

Naloxone will determine the fool in the room. It is this simple. Somebody overdoses. Naloxone will reverse the overdose and prevent death. We need greater access to naloxone. Here the fool will stop all discussion and ask for balance.

Naloxone stops heroin. Naloxone stops fentanyl.

Prescription drug monitoring software does not stop heroin-fentanyl associated mortality.

Less time should be spent asking if we should monitor naloxone and instead we need to discuss the differences between the different naloxone formulations.

Who should be prescribed or when is community naloxone engaged?

- A patient requesting it
- A recent opioid overdose
- A suspected overdose
- Opioid injecting patient
- *Nonmedical* opioid use
- Methadone clinic patient
- Opioid + CNS depressant
- Family 3rd party request
- Residential treatment
- Schools

- After re-entry from jail
- Jail
- After release from 100 % abstinence based clinic
- Geographically distant from emergency care
- CDC pain guideline examples

Modified from *Harm Reduction*

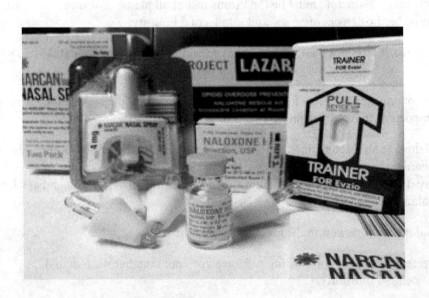

Rethinking Naloxone to fit into the time-line of MAT

Characteristics of Medication Assisted Therapy (MAT)

characteristic	Methadone	Buprenorphine	Naltrexone	Naloxone
Brand Name	Dolophine, Methadose	Subutex, Zusolv, Suboxone	Depade, ReVia, Vivtrol	Narcan, Evzio, Naloxone
Class (schedule)	Agonist (II)	Partial Agonist (III)	Antagonist (none)	Antagonist (none)
Use and Effect	Activates opioid receptor	Activates opioid receptor with diminished response	Blocks opioid receptors and diminishes reward/craving	Blocks opioid receptors and diminishes intrinsic activity
Advantage	• High strength, • Efficacy, • Low cost	• Certified providers reduce need to attend OTP centers; • wider availability	• Not addictive, sedating or doesn't result in dependence; • no special certification; • may be administered by midlevel	• Not addictive, sedating or doesn't result in dependence; • **injection = reversal/ withdrawal;** no special certification; • may be administered by witness/bystander • Low cost options
Disadvantage	Only @ OTP, must visit daily	Measurable abuse risk; **injection = reversal/withdrawal**	Poor oral compliance; induction requires abstinence	Poor oral bioavailability; reduced duration of action
Route	Oral	Sublingual	Oral, I.M.	I.V., I.M., I.N.

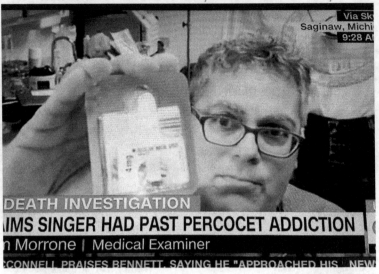

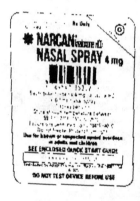

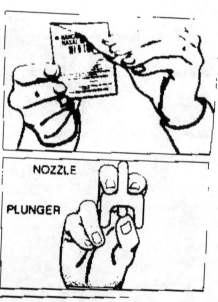

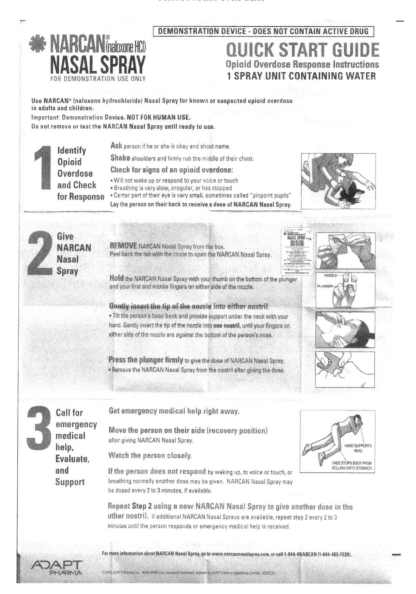

DEMONSTRATION DEVICE - DOES NOT CONTAIN ACTIVE DRUG

✱ NARCAN® (naloxone HCl)
NASAL SPRAY
FOR DEMONSTRATION USE ONLY

QUICK START GUIDE
Opioid Overdose Response Instructions
1 SPRAY UNIT CONTAINING WATER

Use NARCAN® (naloxone hydrochloride) Nasal Spray for known or suspected opioid overdose in adults and children.
Important: Demonstration Device. NOT FOR HUMAN USE.
Do not remove or test the NARCAN Nasal Spray until ready to use.

1 Identify Opioid Overdose and Check for Response

Ask person if he or she is okay and shout name.
Shake shoulders and firmly rub the middle of their chest.
Check for signs of an opioid overdose:
• Will not wake up or respond to your voice or touch
• Breathing is very slow, irregular, or has stopped
• Center part of their eye is very small, sometimes called "pinpoint pupils"
Lay the person on their back to receive a dose of NARCAN Nasal Spray.

2 Give NARCAN Nasal Spray

REMOVE NARCAN Nasal Spray from the box.
Peel back the tab with the circle to open the NARCAN Nasal Spray.

Hold the NARCAN Nasal Spray with your thumb on the bottom of the plunger and your first and middle fingers on either side of the nozzle.

Gently insert the tip of the nozzle into either nostril.
• Tilt the person's head back and provide support under the neck with your hand. Gently insert the tip of the nozzle into one nostril, until your fingers on either side of the nozzle are against the bottom of the person's nose.

Press the plunger firmly to give the dose of NARCAN Nasal Spray.
• Remove the NARCAN Nasal Spray from the nostril after giving the dose.

3 Call for emergency medical help, Evaluate, and Support

Get emergency medical help right away.

Move the person on their side (recovery position) after giving NARCAN Nasal Spray.

Watch the person closely.

If the person does not respond by waking up, to voice or touch, or breathing normally another dose may be given. NARCAN Nasal Spray may be dosed every 2 to 3 minutes, if available.

Repeat Step 2 using a new NARCAN Nasal Spray to give another dose in the other nostril. If additional NARCAN Nasal Sprays are available, repeat step 2 every 2 to 3 minutes until the person responds or emergency medical help is received.

For more information about NARCAN Nasal Spray, go to www.narcannasalspray.com, or call 1-844-4NARCAN (1-844-462-7226).

ADAPT PHARMA

You do not need to prime NARCAN Nasal Spray. use NARCAN Nasal Spray:

Lay the person on their back to receive a dose of NARCAN Nasal Spray. Remove NARCAN Nasal Spray from the box.

Hold the NARCAN Nasal Spray with your thumb on the bottom of the plunger and your first and middle fingers on either side of the nozzle.

Tilt the person's head back and provide support under the neck with your hand. Gently insert the tip of the nozzle into **one nostril** until your fingers on either side of the nozzle are against the bottom of the person's nose.

Press the plunger firmly to give the dose of NARCAN Nasal Spray. Remove the NARCAN Nasal Spray from the nostril after giving the dose.

What to do after NARCAN Nasal Spray has been used: Get emergency medical help right away.

Move the person on their side (recovery position) after giving NARCAN Nasal Spray. Watch the person closely. If the person does not respond by waking up, to voice or touch, or breathing normally another dose may be given. NARCAN Nasal Spray may be dosed every 2 to 3 minutes, if available. Repeat using a new NARCAN Nasal Spray to give another dose in the other nostril. If additional NARCAN Nasal Sprays are available, Steps 2 through 6 may be repeated every 2 to 3 minutes until the person responds or emergency medical help is received.

---

[i] *CDC Health Advisory: Increases in Fentanyl Drug Confiscations and Fentanyl-related Overdose Fatalities. http://emergency.cdc.gov/han/han00384.asp#_edn11*

[ii] *U.S. Drug Enforcement Administration. 21 CFR part 1310. Control of a Chemical Precursor Used in the Illicit Manufacture of Fentanyl as a List 1 Chemical. Federal Register 2007;72:20039—47.*

[iii] *FDA DailyMed prescribing information fentanyl citrate intravenous http://dailymed.nlm.nih.gov/dailymed/drugInfo.cfm?setid=c5d40297-b769-48cc-9f84-f98b7a333507*

[iv] *CDC Health Advisory: Increases in Fentanyl Drug Confiscations and Fentanyl-related Overdose Fatalities. http://emergency.cdc.gov/han/han00384.asp#_edn11*

[v] *Centers for Disease Control and Prevention, National Center for Health Statistics. Multiple Cause of Death" "1999-2014 on CDC WONDER Online Database, released 2015. Data are from the Multiple Cause of Death Files, 1999-2014, as compiled" from data provided by the 57 vital statistics jurisdictions through the Vital Statistics Cooperative Program. Accessed at http://wonder.cdc.gov/mcd-icd10.html on Jan 19, 2016 7:47:47 AM CDC Wonder Database Multiple Cause of Death 2014 UCD - ICD-10 Codes: X40-44; X60-64; X85; Y10-Y14 and MCD – ICD-10 codesT40.1 (Heroin), T40.2 (Other opioids), T40.3 (Methadone), T40.4 (Other synthetic narcotics)*

[vi] *Clinical provision of improvised nasal naloxone without experimental testing and without regulatory approval: imaginative shortcut or dangerous bypass of essential safety procedures? http://onlinelibrary.wiley.com/doi/10.1111/add.13209/full*

[vii] *Addiction 2016: As Heroin Use Escalates, A New Drug To Reverse Overdoses Hits US Drugstores http://www.ibtimes.com/addiction-2016-heroin-use-escalates-new-drug-reverse-overdoses-hits-us-drugstores-2271924*

viii   *FDA Comments on Nasal Naloxone Dose Concerns*
http://www.medpagetoday.com/EmergencyMedicine/EmergencyMedicine/55440

ix   *Summary Review for Regulatory Action*
*http://www.fda.gov/downloads/drugs/developmentapprovalprocess/developmentresources/*ucm4800
92.pdf

x   *http://intranasal.net/OpiateOverdose/Opiate_overdose_overview.htm*

xi   *Dowling et al. Population pharmacokinetics of intravenous, intramuscular, and intranasal naloxone*
in human volunteers. http://www.ncbi.nlm.nih.gov/pubmed/18641540

xii   *Clinical provision of improvised nasal naloxone without experimental testing and without*
regulatory approval: imaginative shortcut or dangerous bypass of essential safety procedures?
http://onlinelibrary.wiley.com/doi/10.1111/add.13209/full

xiii   *US Patent 9,192,570; WO 2015/095644 AntiOp, Inc.*

xiv   *Indivior Receives Complete Response Letter from FDA Not Approving Naloxone Nasal Spray New*
Drug Application for Opioid Overdose http://indivior.com/wp-content/uploads/2015/11/Nasal-
Naloxone-Final-Release_112415.pdf

xv   *Comparative Usability Study of a Novel Auto-Injector and an Intranasal System*
for Naloxone Delivery. http://www.ncbi.nlm.nih.gov/pubmed/25910473

xvi   *Summary Review for Regulatory Action*
*http://www.fda.gov/downloads/drugs/developmentapprovalprocess/developmentresources/*ucm4800
92.pdf

xvii   *Increases in Drug and Opioid Overdose Deaths — United States, 2000–2014*
http://www.cdc.gov/mmwr/preview/mmwrhtml/mm6450a3.htm?s_cid=mm6450a3_w

xviii   *Recommendations for laboratory testing for acetyl fentanyl and patient evaluation and treatment for*
overdose with synthetic opioids http://stacks.cdc.gov/view/cdc/25259

xix   *CDC Health Advisory: Increases in Fentanyl Drug Confiscations and Fentanyl-related Overdose*
Fatalities. http://emergency.cdc.gov/han/han00384.asp#_edn11

xx   *2014 OHIO DRUG OVERDOSE PRELIMINARY DATA: GENERAL FINDINGS*
http://www.healthy.ohio.gov/vipp/data/rxdata.aspx

xxi   *Drug- and Alcohol-Related Intoxication Deaths in Maryland, 2014*
http://bha.dhmh.maryland.gov/OVERDOSE_PREVENTION/SitePages/Data%20and%20Reports.as
px

xxii   *Harvard T.H. Chan School of Public Health Summary of opioid overdose deaths: Massachusetts,*
January – June, 2014 http://s3.amazonaws.com/media.wbur.org/wordpress/15/files/2015/11/Brief-
report-MA-opioid-OD-deaths-2014.pdf

xxiii   *CDC Health Advisory: Increases in Fentanyl Drug Confiscations and Fentanyl-related Overdose*
Fatalities. http://emergency.cdc.gov/han/han00384.asp#_edn11

xxiv   *Rhode Island's Strategic Plan on Addiction and Overdose*
http://www.health.ri.gov/news/temp/RhodeIslandsStrategicPlanOnAddictionAndOverdose.pdf

xxv   *Maine Attorney General August 20 2015. http://www.maine.gov/ag/news/article.shtml?id=653671*

xxvi   *THIS IS AN OFFICIAL NH DHHS HEALTH ALERT*
http://www.dhhs.nh.gov/dphs/cdcs/alerts/documents/opioid.pdf

xxvii   *Analysis of Drug-Related Overdose Deaths in Pennsylvania, 2014*
http://www.dea.gov/divisions/phi/2015/phi111715_attach.pdf

xxviii   *Connecticut Office of Chief Medical Examiner*
http://www.ct.gov/ocme/lib/ocme/AccidentalDrugIntoxication2015.pdf

xxix   *OVERDOSE DEATHS INVOLVING FENTANYL UP DRAMATICALLY IN DELAWARE*
http://dhss.delaware.gov/dhss/pressreleases/2015/fentanyldeaths-122815.html

xxx   *Drug Related Fatalities Vermont Department of Health*
http://healthvermont.gov/research/documents/databrief_drug_related_fatalities.pdf

xxxi   *Fatal Drug Overdose Quarterly Report Virginia Department of Health*
https://www.google.ie/url?sa=t&rct=j&q=&esrc=s&source=web&cd=4&cad=rja&uact=8&ved=
0ahUKEwjxicLYiPzKAhUCPQ8KHTvHAMMQFgguMAM&url=https%3A%2F%2Fwww.vdh.virgin
ia.gov%2FmedExam%2Fdocuments%2Fpdf%2FQuarterly%2520Drug%2520Death%2520Report.p
df&usg=AFQjCNGdcVORWdMwp2WhYoaXCZlEBSSopg&sig2=vOseqo73p9iTIPAXJNFNAA

xxxii   *http://www.ems1.com/naloxone/articles/11079048-Chicago-medics-treat-74-narcotics-overdoses-in-72-hours/*

xxxiii   *http://dirtyjerseyrecovery.com/2014/06/nj-news-shore-program-countering-heroin-overdoses-going-state-wide/*

xxxiv   *http://mobile.buffalonews.com/?articleRedirect=1&url=http%3A%2F%2F-*
www.buffalonews.com%2Fcity-region%2F23-dead-in-erie-county-from-opiates-over-11-days-20160209

ADDENDUM #1.

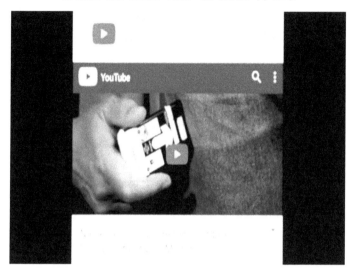

https://m.youtube.com/watch?v=yKmOZR6WefU

Heroin and Fentanyl Co-flation

- Millions of people (not thousands) are using heroin. Its not getting better. Looking at Rx opioids is very 5 years ago.
- The number of state and federal overdose deaths is grossly in error (low) for many institutional reasons.
- The poor will die on the street and in libraries.
- The working will die at home (60%) and work (30%).
- The young will die at home, schools and restaurants.
- Hospitals, societies and medical schools are equally as guilty as Big Pharma because they refused to accept addiction medicine & they perpetuated stigma.
- Grant money to help goes to the same megalithic dinosaurs that have no new ideas. They only self perpetuate.
- Naloxone should fall like rain. 1,000,000 doctors are blind.

ADDENDUM #2.

OPIOID ANTAGONIST: STANDING ORDER RX

H.B. 5326 (S-1): SUMMARY OF BILL REPORTED FROM COMMITTEE

Senate Fiscal Agency
P. O. Box 30036
Lansing, Michigan 48909-7536

BILL ANALYSIS

Telephone: (517) 373-5383
Fax: (517) 373-1986

House Bill 5326 (Substitute S-1 as reported)

House Committee: Health Policy Senate Committee: Health Policy

———

The bill would amend the Public Health Code to do the following regarding opioid antagonists:

Include in the definition of "prescription" a standing order for an opioid antagonist issued by the chief medical executive of the State.

Allow the chief medical executive to issue a standing order that did not identify a particular patient for the purpose of dispensing opioid antagonists to individuals.

Allow a pharmacist to dispense an opioid antagonist to any individual pursuant to the standing order.

Provide that the chief medical executive, or pharmacist who dispensed an opioid antagonist as authorized under the bill, would not be liable in a civil action for damages resulting from the dispensing of the opioid antagonist or the administration of or the failure to administer an opioid antagonist.

Require the Department of Licensing and Regulatory Affairs, in conjunction

68

with the Department of Health and Human Services (DHHS), to promulgate rules to implement these provisions.

Require a reference to the standing order to be included on a receipt furnished to the purchaser of the prescription drug. The bill also would do the following with regard to an annual inventory of Schedule 2 through 5 controlled substances conducted by a person licensed to manufacture, distribute, prescribe, or dispense controlled substances:

Delete a requirement that the person submit a report of the inventory to the Michigan Board of Pharmacy.

Eliminate a $25,000 civil fine for a violation of the inventory requirements.

Require the person to retain the inventory for at least two years and make it available for inspection by DHHS upon request. Additionally, the bill would do the following in relation to the State's controlled substances electronic monitoring system:

Eliminate a December 31, 2016, sunset on a provision allowing the DHHS Director toshare data from the system with a health care payment or benefit provider.

Reenact a provision that expired on February 1, 2016, allowing DHHS to issue a request to a health care payment or benefit provider to determine how many times the provider accessed the system in the previous year.

Eliminate a requirement that the Controlled Substances Advisory Commission include in its annual report on its activities and recommendations information on the system's implementation and effectiveness.

Page 1 of 2 hb5326/1516

The bill also would establish an effective date of January 1, 2020, for continuing education requirements applicable to a licensee seeking renewal of a veterinarian's or veterinary technician's license.

MCL 333.7333a et al. Legislative Analyst: Julie Cassidy

FISCAL IMPACT

The bill would have an indeterminate, but likely minor fiscal impact on the Department of Licensing and Regulatory Affairs (LARA), and local units of government.

Under the bill, LARA would be required to promulgate rules regarding the implementation of a standing order for opioid antagonists.

The cost to promulgate rules would depend largely on their complexity, and those costs would be borne by existing LARA resources.

Additionally, the bill would have an **indeterminate fiscal impact** on the Department of Health and Human Services.

Opioid antagonists are covered under the State's Medicaid program.

To the extent that the bill would increase use of these prescription drugs, the State would face increased costs.

If increased access to opioid antagonists resulted in a reduction in covered visits to hospitals for treatment of the effects of a drug overdose, the State would see a potential reduction in Medicaid costs that could partially or completely offset the costs related to increased use.

The same cost impacts also would be reflected in health care costs for State and local governmental employees.

The bill also would remove a civil fine for failing to keep an annual inventory of all Schedule 2 to 5 controlled substances.

Date Completed: 11-30-16 Fiscal Analyst: Ellyn Ackerman Ryan Bergan

Floor\hb5326 This analysis was prepared by nonpartisan Senate staff for use by the Senate in its deliberations and does not constitute an official statement of legislative intent.

Page 2 of 2 Bill Analysis @ www.senate.michigan.gov/sfa hb5326/1516

ADDENDUM #3.

Joint Position Statements of the American Psychiatric Association and the American Academy of Addiction Psychiatry : Opioid Overdose Education and Naloxone Distribution, PA Standing Order & AOAAM naloxone white paper

Approved by the Board of Trustees, December 2015

Approved by the Assembly, November 2015

"Policy documents are approved by the APA Assembly and Board of Trustees. . . These are . . . position statements that define APA official policy on specific subjects. . ." – APA Operations Manual

Issue: There has been a significant increase in mortality from prescription drug overdoses over the past 20 years in the U.S. (1). Overdose deaths now exceed automobile accidents as the leading preventable cause of death by injury in the U.S., posing a significant public health crisis (2). Rates of opioid overdose have surged throughout the world, including in Canada, Europe, Asia, and Australia (3-7). In addition to the traditional risks associated with heroin use, increasing use of opioid analgesics (especially long-acting formulations at high doses) has been a major contributor to increased overdose mortality (8-10).

APA POSITION:

The American Psychiatric Association and the American Academy of Addiction Psychiatry endorse expanded access to naloxone, along with appropriate training and education, for bystanders, family members, and other individuals who may be in a position to initiate early response to opioid overdose, including EMTs, paramedics, corrections officers, and law enforcement. Naloxone kits should be distributed to individuals at high risk of witnessing or experiencing an opioid overdose, including users of heroin or other opioid drugs. Additionally, naloxone should be prescribed to groups at heightened risk for opioid-induced respiratory depression including individuals: 1) on high-dose full-agonist opioid pharmacotherapy (i.e. greater than 100 mg of morphine equivalence per day), 2) prescribed opioids in combination with benzodiazepines, and/or 3) suspected or known nonmedical opioid use (15).

Individuals authorized to dispense naloxone overdose kits should be required to undergo training and education in the recognition of signs and symptoms of overdose, techniques for administration of naloxone, and referral to emergency medical services. Supervision and training of these individuals should be maintained on an ongoing basis.

Additionally, states should actively protect the efforts of providers and civilians through Good Samaritan laws, amnesty protections for certified providers, and the allowance of third-party prescriptions (i.e. for the family member of the index patient). States with limitations on access to naloxone should be encouraged by their state health officials and medical societies to broaden distribution of naloxone and support legislation to remove barriers to naloxone access.

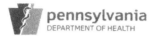

STANDING ORDER DOH-002-2016

Naloxone Prescription for Overdose Prevention

Naloxone Hydrochloride (Naloxone) is a medication indicated for reversal of opioid overdose in the event of a drug overdose that is the result of consumption or use of one or more opioid-related drugs causing a drug overdose event.

I. PURPOSE

This standing order is intended to ensure that residents of the Commonwealth of Pennsylvania who are at risk of experiencing an opioid-related overdose, or who are family members, friends or other persons who are in a position to assist a person at risk of experiencing an opioid-related overdose (Eligible Persons), are able to obtain Naloxone. This order is not intended to be used by organizations who employ or contract with medical staff who are authorized to write prescriptions. Such organizations should utilize the medical professionals with whom they have a relationship to write prescriptions specific to personnel who would be expected to administer Naloxone, and would be wise to ensure that all such personnel are appropriately trained in the administration of Naloxone.

II. AUTHORITY

This standing order is issued pursuant to Act 139 of 2014 (Act 139) (amending The Controlled Substance, Drug, Device and Cosmetic Act (35 P.S. §§ 780-101 et seq.)), which permits health care professionals otherwise authorized to prescribe Naloxone to prescribe it via standing order to Eligible Persons.

III. AUTHORIZATION

This standing order may be used by Eligible Persons as a prescription or third-party prescription to obtain Naloxone from a pharmacy in the event that they are unable to obtain Naloxone or a prescription for Naloxone from their regular health care providers or another source. This order is authorization for pharmacists to dispense Naloxone and devices for its administration SOLELY in the forms prescribed herein.

IV. TRAINING AND INSTRUCTIONAL MATERIALS

Prior to obtaining Naloxone under this standing order, Eligible Persons are strongly advised to complete a training program approved by the Pennsylvania Department of Health (DOH) in consultation with the Pennsylvania Department of Drug and Alcohol Programs (DDAP), such as the one found on line at http://www.getnaloxonenow.org/online_training.html or at the DOH

1 | NALOXONE STANDING ORDER-DOH-002

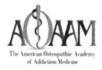

Use of Naloxone - Prevention of Opioid Overdose Deaths

The abuse of, and addiction to, opioids is a serious and challenging public health problem. Deaths from drug overdose have risen steadily over the past two decades and are now the leading cause of injury death in the United States   Prescription opioid analgesics, e.g. hydrocodone, oxycodone, morphine, and methadone, used to treat both acute and chronic pain, have increasingly been implicated in drug overdose deaths over the last decade. From 1999 to 2013, the rate of drug poisoning deaths involving opioid analgesics nearly quadrupled.

Deaths related to heroin have also increased sharply since 2010, resulting in a 39 percent increase between 2012 and 2013. Given these alarming trends, we need to be an intellectually honest, sustainable, and transparent, discussion concerning the prevention, identification and treatment of individuals with an opioid use disorder. Included in this discussion there needs to be an understanding of the utility of naloxone in the prevention of opioid overdose deaths. As an opioid antagonist, naloxone is an effective medication in blocking opioid receptor activation thus reversing opioid overdose.

It can, if given soon enough, restore normal respirations in a person whose breathing has slowed or stopped as a result of heroin or prescription opioid overdose.

Several overdose education and naloxone distribution programs have been developed to provide instruction on its use and direct issuing of the medication to opioid users, associates, and families. These programs are attempting to get it into the hands of anyone that may have a potential of being in the presence of someone using opioids at risk of overdose. This includes those prescribed opioids for pain that are either concurrently prescribed a sedative hypnotic medication or on high dose opioids, and those with a history of alcohol and other drug use problems.

The Center for Disease Control reported that between 1996 and 2010 more than 10,000 overdose reversals took place nationwide as a result of the distribution of naloxone to nonmedical personnel. As of November 2014, 23 states have statutes that allow for "third-party" prescriptions of naloxone.

This allows for the prescription to be written for a person other than the person that may receive the medication such as a friend, relative or person in a position to assist a person at risk of experiencing an opioid overdose. An evaluation of Massachusetts' overdose education and nasal naloxone distribution program found that opioid overdose death rates declined in communities where programs were implemented compared to those where it was not available.

The FDA is also supporting the development of new opioid overdose treatments by using expedited review programs. Given the effectiveness of naloxone in overdose reversal, the Food and Drug Administration (FDA) has encouraged innovations in more user-friendly naloxone delivery systems such as auto-injectors, made particularly for lay use outside of health care settings.

The American Osteopathic Academy of Addiction Medicine supports the important role of naloxone, an opioid antagonist plays in overdose prevention. This AOAAM policy focuses on five objectives.

The AOAAM will:

1. **Expand our support** in media, curriculum and CME to advocate for responsible utilization of naloxone in overdose prevention.

2. **Partner with other individuals and organizations** to advance the awareness of naloxone in the prevention of opioid overdose by the media, state and federal governments, health care providers and the public.

3. **Encourage further grant support and public policy** that underwrites the distribution of naloxone.

4. **Offer our experience and expertise** to government, research, education and industry in their efforts to accelerate the development and availability of naloxone and user-friendly delivery systems. .

5. AOAAM will make every effort to identify, **create, and disseminate best practice naloxone or antagonist delivery models and strategies** to all stakeholders.

ADDENDUM #4.

Who supports community naloxone??

- White House
- ONDCP
- HHS
- SAMHSA
- CDC
- NIH & NIDA
- DoD
- VA
- WHO

- Fort Bragg, NC
- Johns Hopkins
- Harvard University
- Boston University
- Temple University
- University of Michigan
- ACP
- AMA
- ASAM
- FSMB

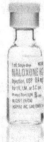

ADDENDUM #5.

Timely Naloxone has reversed fentanyl associated anesthesia in hospitals for decades. It is the only hope in Heroin-Fentanyl associated mortality

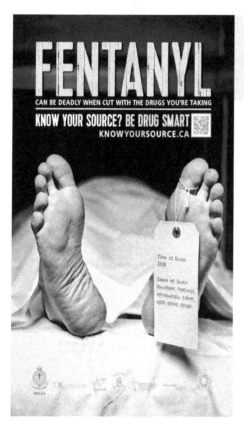

Pharmacology

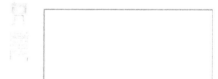

Rational prescribing will not translate 1st order impact to heroin overdose deaths

MAT will impact OD & we need the 275 limit

Naloxone will impact OD most directly

ADDENDUM #6.

Autoinjectors, Naloxone Access User's Guide Assembly, Nasal Narcan Activation and assorted naloxone pharmacokinetics

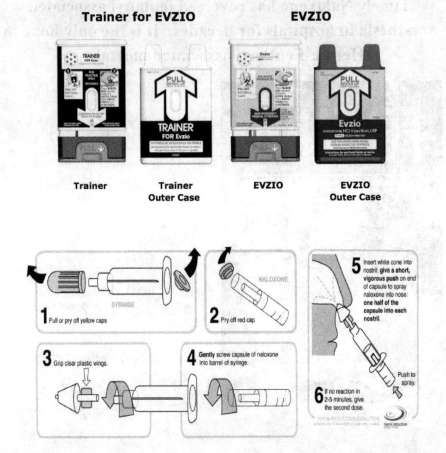

Improvised nasal naloxone assembly from components including (mucosal atomizer device) MAD

Spray pattern of Nasal Narcan, one dose, no neeedle.

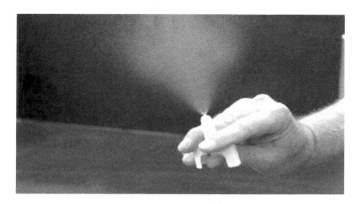

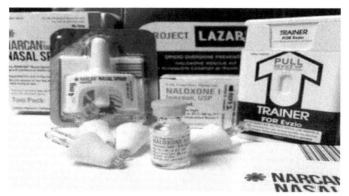

Naloxone Formulations-Pharmacokinetics

Route	Dose	C_{max} (pg/mL)	T_{max} (hr)	AUC1-hr (hr-pg/mL)	$t_{1/2}$ (hr)	Ref
IV	0.036 mg/kg	26270 ± 11890*	0.05	12730 ± 2550*	NR	1
IN	20 mg Crushed Powder	20180 ± 5710*	0.28	29830 ± 12470*	NR	1
IN	**4 mg (NARCAN) ***	**4830 (43.1%)**	**0.5**	**7980 (37.3%)**	**2.08 (29.8%)**	2
IM	2 mg (Syringe)	4160 (43.9%)	0.25	8088 (13.5%)	1.47 (24.2%)	3
IN	2 mg (Off label kit)	1163 (47.6%)	0.25	1411 (36.7%)	1.44 (17.2%)	3
IM/SC	**0.4 mg (EVZIO) ***	**1100 (52.4%)**	**0.25**	**1880 (24.7%)**	**1.22 (28.2%)**	4
IM/SC	0.4 mg (Syringe)	857 (53.2%)	0.33	1910 (27.5%)	1.32 (22%)	4
IN	2 mg+ oxy (Off label kit)	871 (48.9%)	0.33	1077 (36.3%)	1.48 (20.7%)	3

* Data presented as mean ± SD. Other data presented as geometric mean (gCV%); Ref # 3 oxy is decongestant oxymetazoline.

79

ADDENDUM #7.

12 Counties in Michigan offer community naloxone and law enforcement naloxone (2017). Intra-state naloxone remains "fractured" all across America.

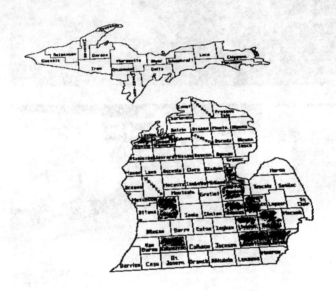

ADDENDUM #8.

ASAM Naloxone press release circa 2014

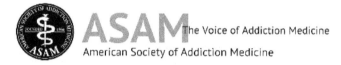

ASAM The Voice of Addiction Medicine
American Society of Addiction Medicine

FOR IMMEDIATE RELEASE
Contact: Alexis Geier Horan, ageier@asam.org, 202-276-7873

ASAM Revises Public Policy Statement on the Use of Naloxone for the Prevention of Drug Overdose Deaths

CHEVY CHASE, MD, SEPTEMBER 11, 2014 – The American Society of Addiction Medicine (ASAM) has updated its Public Policy Statement on the Use of Naloxone for the Prevention of Drug Overdose Deaths. Specifically, the revision recommends the employment of "co-prescription" programs in which prescriptions for naloxone could be prescribed simultaneously with prescriptions for high-potency opioids and that all addiction treatment agencies have on-site supplies of naloxone for "rescue" dosing. The revision also recommends that all jurisdictions adopt laws that would offer naloxone providers and users immunity from prosecution and/or civil liability.

"Expanding access to naloxone should be part of any strategy attempting to reduce the morbidity and mortality associated with opioid addiction" offers Dr. Stuart Gitlow, ASAM President. "The use of naloxone to reverse opioid overdose not only saves lives but also provides an opportunity to engage the addicted individual in treatment."

The revised policy statement maintains its recommendations that naloxone recipients also receive education in the prevention, detection and appropriate response to drug overdose and that research into the identification of new opioid antagonists and/or delivery systems continue.

The Public Needs to Know

Opioid addiction is a chronic disease and is treatable with stabilizing medications, psychosocial interventions and recovery support programs. Even so, millions of Americans currently in need of treatment are unable to access it. ASAM is an association of physicians and associated professionals dedicated to improving the treatment of alcohol, drug and other addictions, educating physicians and medical students, promoting research and prevention, and enlightening and informing the medical community and the public about these issues.

For more information regarding addiction treatment and to access ASAM's public policy statements, please visit www.asam.org.

81

ADDENDUM #9.

*FDA, CDC, NIDA and HHS Public Meeting Naloxone Uptake press release
(2012)*

MEETING HIGHLIGHTS

Role of Naloxone in Opioid Overdose Fatality Prevention Post Meeting Summary

Naloxone is an opioid receptor antagonist that is approved for use by injection only for the reversal of opioid overdose and for adjunct use in the treatment of septic shock. It is currently being used mainly in emergency departments and in ambulances by trained medical professionals. There have been efforts to expand its use by providing the drug to some patients with take-home opioid prescriptions and those who inject illicit drugs, potentially facilitating earlier administration of the drug. On April 12, 2012, FDA, CDC, NIDA and the HHS Office of the Assistant Secretary for Health sponsored a public meeting to initiate a discussion about whether naloxone should be made more widely available outside of conventional medical settings. A link to the meeting page that contains additional information is located here: http://www.fda.gov/Drugs/NewsEvents/ucm277119.htm.

Meeting Highlights

The White House Office of National Drug Control Policy (ONDCP) Prescription Drug Abuse Prevention Plan includes a discussion of naloxone. A statement on behalf of ONDCP Director, Gil Kerlikowske, was read at the meeting. It noted that the Obama Administration recognizes "the important role naloxone can play in overcoming drug overdoses," as articulated its 2010 National Drug Control Strategic Plan.

In the United States, mortality rates closely correlate with opioid sales. In 2008, approximately 36,450 people died from drug overdoses. At least 14,800 of these deaths involved prescription opioid analgesics. Moreover, according to the Substance Abuse and Mental Health Services Administration, the number/rate of Americans 12 years of age and older who currently abuse pain relievers has increased by 20 percent between 2002 and 2009.

The UN Commission on Narcotics Drugs "encourages all Member States to include effective elements for the prevention and treatment of drug overdose, in particular opioid overdose, in national drug policies, where appropriate, and to share best practices and information on the prevention and treatment of drug overdose, in particular opioid overdose, including the use of opioid receptor antagonists such as naloxone."

Most speakers agreed that there should be easier access to naloxone. One speaker said that better data are needed on whether naloxone is effective in saving lives. One issue to be addressed is the relatively short half-life of naloxone compared to some longer-acting opioid formulations. After naloxone is administered, it is important to seek immediate medical attention.

Speakers commented on the concern that increasing the overall availability of naloxone might lead to increased drug use by giving a false sense of security, and suggested this was not a likely concern.

An overview of research related to attitudes and behaviors related to STDs, and in particular to HPV vaccination (Gardasil), presented at the meeting reported no association with an increase in unprotected sex among sexually active women. Similarly, no evidence for greater risk-taking has been seen in the area of protective equipment to prevent childhood injuries (such as bike helmets).

One speaker said that such interventions do not necessarily lead to more risky behaviors. Instead, the results are dependent on the prevention strategy, the target of the strategy, individual characteristics and the larger social context.

Most speakers participating in the open public hearing, some of whom had lost family members or friends to opioid overdose, recommended that the use of naloxone be switched to over-the-counter (OTC) status and encouraged FDA to quickly take steps to improve access to the drug, including by approving non- injectable forms (e.g., intranasal) of the drug.

FDA discussed the general pathways to expand access to naloxone through the development of new formulations or making naloxone approved for use over the counter (OTC).

Gaining FDA approval for a new naloxone formulation, such as an intranasal or auto-injector form, would require a bioequivalence study. In such a trial, drug levels with the new and injectable forms of naloxone would be compared. Such studies typically require fewer than 100 subjects. Data related to safety, chemistry and manufacturing as well as data related to the device used to administer the drug are necessary.

Switching naloxone to over the counter would likely require additional clinical data that answers the following questions:

Can patients (or caregivers) understand directions?
Can patients (or caregivers) follow directions?
Can patients (or caregivers) properly decide if they should use the product?

In addition, data would need to be collected on the new naloxone product to see if OTC consumers are able to use it safely.

Speakers agreed that there is a need for better coordination among Federal agencies, manufacturers and other stakeholder groups to resolve regulatory issues and improve access to the drug.

The meeting ended with each of the Federal partners expressing a willingness to work with interested manufacturers and developers to further explore the best uses of naloxone to prevent opioid overdose deaths.

ADDENDUM #10.

City and County of SanFrancisco Naloxone Policy, Department of Public Health -
October 30, 2013 - Community Behavioral Health Sciences Community Oriented Primary
Care San Francisco General Hospital

Edwin M Lee, Mayor - Take Home Naloxone

Primary care clinics will be prescribing take-home naloxone for patients at risk for opioid overdose, this
includes patients on long term opioids for pain and those abusing prescription opioids or heroin.
Formulations: naloxone can be given by intramuscular (IM) injection or intranasal (IN) administration.
Most patients will be prescribed IN naloxone because it is equally effective and more convenient.

Intramuscular	Intranasal
Naloxone 0.4mg/ml single dose vial, 2 vials NDC # 00409-1215-01 SIG: Inject 1 ml IM upon signs of opioid overdose. Call 911. May repeat x 1. **Syringe 3ml 22G X 1 1/2" # 2** SIG: Use as directed for naloxone administration.	**Naloxone 2mg/2ml prefilled syringe, 2 syringes** NDC # 76329-3369-01 SIG: Spray one-half of syringe into each nostril upon signs of opioid overdose. Call 911. May repeat x 1. (Atomizers will be given to patients in clinic. Please verify the patient has received the atomizer before picking up prescription.)

Patient Counseling: naloxone is a bystander administered drug which means family and
caregivers should be included in patient counseling. If they are not available then the patient
should be instructed to train others in case of an overdose. **Billing and Formulary Status:**
Naloxone vials and prefilled syringes are covered by all local health plans including Healthy
San Francisco, San Francisco Mental Health Plan, and MediCal. For the MediCal HMO plans
naloxone is a "carve-out" medication. This means that claims will have to be submitted
directly to FFS MediCal. Do not send PA requests to the MediCal HMO health plans. Most
Medicare plans also cover both formulations of naloxone.

More information: PRESCRIBETOPREVENT.ORG

ADDENDUM #11.

Midwestern Heroin Sprawl

**Unintentional Poisoning ED visits and Hospitalization
for Opiates and other Narcotics
Dane County, 2007-2011**

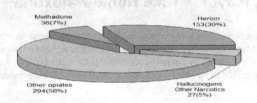

*Heroin accounts for 3 out of 10 autopsied deaths from Substance Use
Disorder on toxicology in Central Wisconsin (2007-2011).*

Midland Drug Choice on admission to treatment (MDCH/Fast Ice*)

Midland	2014	2015	2016*
alcohol	39%	30%	15%
All opioid	53%	63%	83%
Rx opioid	29%	29%	21%
HEROIN	**24%**	**34%**	**62%**

*Heroin accounts for 6 out of 10 admissions to outpatient Substance Use
Disorder Diagnosis on admission in CMH for (Midland, Michigan) Central
Michigan (2016).*

ADDENDUM #12.

Drugs or alcohol have been questioned in the news with the deaths of many American celebrities. Even prescription drugs re-wire the brain and people do things that they would never have done.

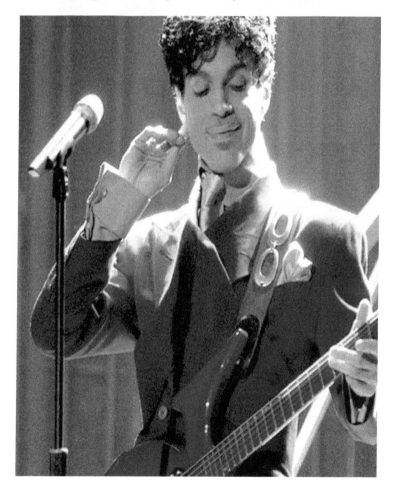

Prince

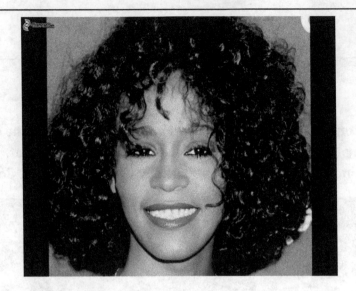

Houston

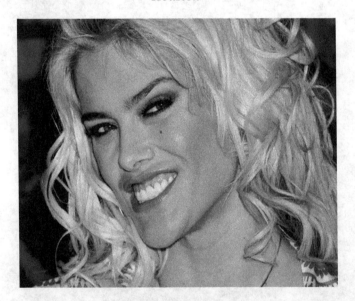

Smith

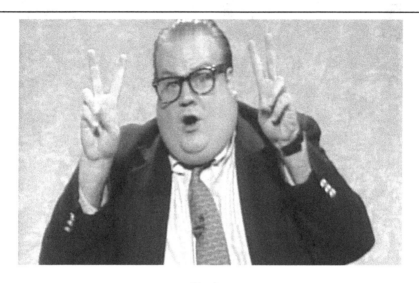

Farley

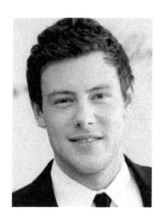

Corey

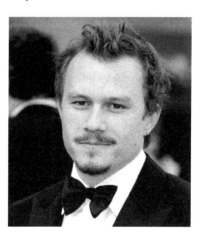

Ledger

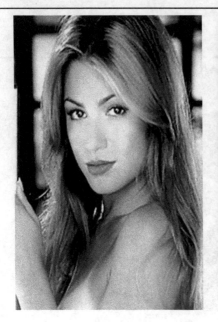

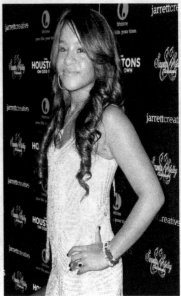

Bridges   *Brown*

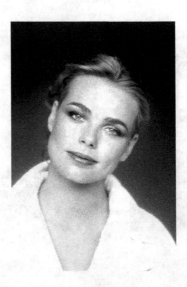

Hemmingway

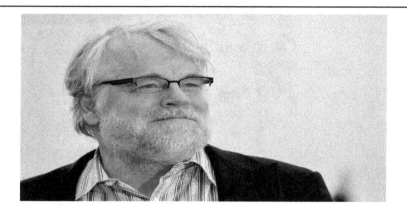

Hoffman

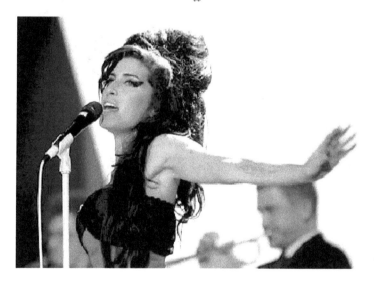

Winehouse

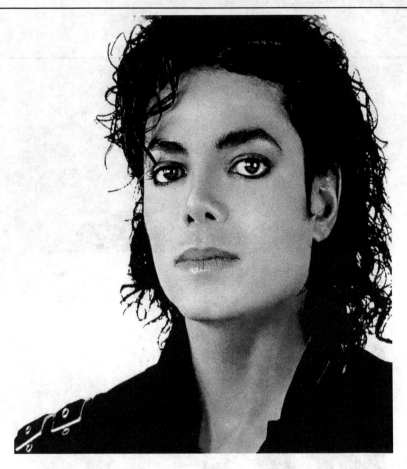

Jackson

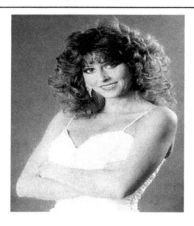

Miss Elizabeth

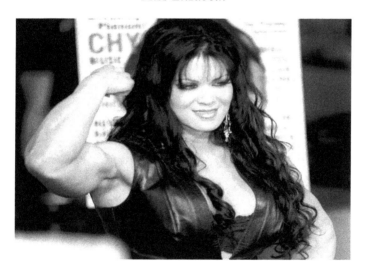

Chyna

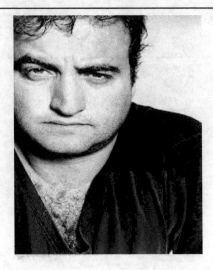

Belushi

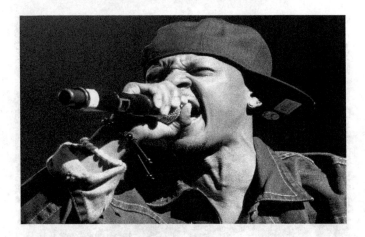

Chris Cross

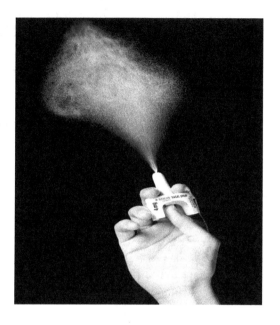

FDA approved one dose needless Nasal Narcan (naloxone) 4mg/0.1mL spray

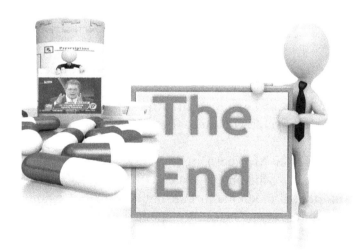

William Morrone, DO, MPH, MS, FAOAAM, ASAM, FACOFP, DABAM and DAAPM, is Family and Community Medicine faculty, at The Michigan State University College of Osteopathic Medicine (MSUCOM), and has been Asst Director of Family Medicine at Synergy/CMU and a liaison in the Department of Psychiatry. He is author of *American Narcan*, America's first book on community naloxone & heroin-fentanyl associated mortality. Dr. Morrone founded Overdose Recovery Radio and he goes into jail to start drug treatment.

He has been a village physician in Huron County and his addiction clinics serve 37 counties and 52 zip codes. He is triple board certified by the American Board of Addiction Medicine, American College of Osteopathic Family Practitioners and the American Academy of Pain Management. Dr. Morrone was a Ruth Fox faculty for the 42nd ASAM Conference in Washington DC and is an active addiction educator, social advocate in pain management and has contributed numerous didactic pieces on heroin, naloxone, opioids, overdoses, REMS, drug court and naltrexone to 17 state medical and national societies. His CNN international analysis of the 2016 Prince overdose related death was seen by *100 million* people world-wide.

He also holds an MPH and a *graduate degree in toxicology and pharmacology* from the University of Missouri at Kansas City, graduate school of pharmacy. Most notable to *pop culture cable TV news viewers* is that he has been the *"forensic toxicologist"* on PrimeTime Justice with Ashleigh Banfield, Nancy Grace-CNN/HLN, Court TV, CNN, FOXNews Channel and MSNBC giving medical opinions on drug addiction or death and the 6 stages of decomposition. Public service is no stranger to Dr. Morrone, as he is a Deputy Chief Medical Examiner, a Diplomat of American College of Forensic Examiners and has been a volunteer firefighter.

Dr. Morrone has been Medical Director at Queen of Angels Detox and HoM Hospice. Dr. Morrone graduated from MSUCOM, served his internship in internal medicine in Lansing at Ingham Regional Medical Center and his residency in family medicine at the Michigan State University COM statewide campus site in Bay City.

http://www.DrMorrone.com

CPSIA information can be obtained
at www.ICGtesting.com
Printed in the USA
BVHW032138121022
649352BV00010B/277